Dr Ross Walker is an eminent cardiologist with a passion for people and health. He graduated from the University of New South Wales with Honours in 1979 and became a Fellow of the Royal Australasian College of Physicians (FRACP) in 1986. His special interests are advanced echocardiology and preventative cardiology. He is the author of the best-selling books *If I Eat Another Carrot I'll Go Crazy*, *What's Cookin' Doc*, *Highway to Health*, *The Cell Factor* and *The Life Factor*, all concentrating on lifestyle issues and in particular diet, antioxidants and health.

Dr Walker lectures extensively throughout the world to medical and business groups. He often discusses health and stress in the Australian media and has a weekly program on Radio 3AW in Melbourne and a monthly show on Radio 2CH in Sydney, in which he discusses preventative health issues.

He lives in Sydney and is married with five children.

www.drrosswalker.com
www.thefordhamcompany.com.au

Also by Ross Walker and available from Pan Macmillan

The Cell Factor
The Life Factor

DIETS DON'T WORK

A cardiologist's real program for losing weight permanently, staying healthy and living longer

DR ROSS WALKER
M.B., B.S. (HONS), F.R.A.C.P

MACMILLAN
Pan Macmillan Australia

To my brother, Ian

First published in 2006 by Pan Macmillan Australia Pty Limited
1 Market Street, Sydney

Reprinted 2006

National Library of Australia
Cataloguing-in-Publication data:

Walker, Ross G.T.
Diets don't work: a cardiologist's real program for losing weight permanently, staying healthy and living longer.

ISBN 978 1 40503 715 0.

ISBN 1 40503715 6.

1. Health attitudes. 2. Reducing diets. 3. Exercise.
I. Title

613.2

Papers used by Pan Macmillan Australia Pty Ltd are natural, recyclable products made from wood grown in sustainable forests. The manufacturing processes conform to the environmental regulations of the country of origin.

Set in 11.5/16.5 pt Sabon by Midland Typesetters, Australia
Printed in Australia by McPherson's Printing Group

Contents

Introduction

Most people reading this book, indeed most people living in our modern Western world, have been involved in an experiment. This experiment has gone sadly and horribly wrong. What am I referring to? Diets!

Diet books abound, but to no avail. Look around any street or shopping mall and you can see that diets are not working. Despite being bombarded with the dieting message for the past 20 to 30 years, people are getting fatter and are more tired. Society is overwhelmed by the modern diseases of obesity, heart disease, diabetes and cancer.

The major aim of this book is to act as a reminder – our bodies were designed to exist in a natural environment, not in our modern, synthetic, fast-paced world. So the best way to be healthy and to achieve and maintain an ideal weight is to eat and live as naturally as we can.

Part 1 explains the many reasons for our current health and stress problems. To understand these, it is important to be aware of how human beings started out. I will examine our early origins as 'hunter-gatherers' and make the vital point that we haven't evolved far from this natural physiology, which existed around the simple experiences of feast, famine and constant movement.

In our modern world, because of the abundant food supply, the availability of forms of transport other than our legs and the increasingly sedentary nature of our work and play, we are overwhelming our once-efficient fat storage mechanisms, which were designed to tide us over the now nonexistent times of famine. We are surrounded by synthetic chemicals, and we have developed a complex, stressful life with a profound dependence on technology, without much scope for flexibility.

The benefit of modern living is that it enables us to satisfy most of our needs easily and efficiently. This gives us time to do other things, but at a cost: we are more readily bored, we inadvertently miss or skip activities that we need (such as exercise and properly prepared meals), and we damage ourselves with unnatural chemicals, deficiencies and stress.

One thing I am certain of is that convenience is killing us.

Convenience has led to assault upon our bodies by free radicals. Two major contributors to this are our excessive exposure to synthetic chemicals and the ubiquitous presence of chronic stress. Free radicals, if unchecked, oxidise and damage our cells and metabolic processes, leading to disease. If we consider our bodies as an invaded country, the free radicals are the 'bad guys' and our cells are individual castles defending us against their invasion.

After 25 years of practising cardiology, I have treated thousands of patients, and have witnessed the burgeoning pharmaceutical therapies and the arrival of technologies and interventions to treat all manner of diseases. It is obvious to me that these modern treatments provide only a partial answer. We are living longer, but I do not believe we are living better.

I have two distinct groups of patients. The first are content to follow the modern line of thinking – 'I'll have the operation' or 'I'll swallow the pills' – without changing anything in their lifestyle or diet. Unfortunately, this is the norm, not the exception. I watch these patients progressively block their arteries and whittle away bits of their heart and brain, and often their toes, feet and legs.

The second type of patient are people who might have symptoms or even need major surgery but, either way, they decide to follow the Dr Walker Lifestyle Program – not for 12 weeks but for the rest of their lives – with the result that they keep on keeping on (to borrow that battery ad phrase). Part 2 offers advice on preventing and overcoming attack by free radicals by eating and living as naturally as possible in the modern world, involving an introduction to body types and their origins in distinct geographic characteristics.

Part 3 acknowledges that although there is a general need for us to return to a more natural way of life, once we have achieved this, there is still important fine-tuning that can allow us to experience optimum health. This fine-tuning is centred on the concept that 'one size does not fit all'. I will explain how body types determine the best eating and living plans for individuals.

The Dr Walker Lifestyle Program will help you to attain your ideal body weight. On reaching this point, lifelong maintenance should be your goal, and this is where the body type advice will guide you towards long-term optimum health.

PART 1

HUNTER-GATHERER VS MODERN WESTERN SOCIETY

CHAPTER 1

Convenience is killing us

Picture the scene. It is 6 a.m. in Bedrock Quays, the latest in resort-style living for the prehistoric set, and an alarm clock sounds (well, sounds is probably stretching things a bit far – the alarm is more likely the reflection off a sundial, or a bird crowing about the fact that it has evolved wings). Our hero, Hunter-Gatherer Man (let's call him H-G for convenience), drags himself off his not-so-comfortable bed on the floor of his designer cave, has a breakfast of nuts and berries, forgets to shave (because he doesn't own a razor and shaving hasn't been invented yet), puts on the latest fashion in bearskin and wanders off to start another hard slog in Jungles-R-Us. Hopefully, he will snare a tasty animal to feed his wife and offspring.

Sometimes he is successful, sometimes he is not. But he knows his job – to ensure the survival of his family and himself.

At a very basic level, the function of every organism is to survive, and everything in nature survives in a natural system. Human beings were designed as hunter-gatherers, and as a part of the environment. A major factor in hunter-gatherer eating patterns was availability, and since fresh, natural food decays very rapidly once caught or collected, it had to be consumed immediately. Therefore, if the hunter-gatherers killed a wild animal, there was no storing the carcass in the prehistoric Kelvinator; they either ate it or wasted it. On the other hand, if there was no food to be found, then the hunter-gatherers didn't eat.

This pattern of feast and famine was the experience of ancient humans throughout their lives. If they were wandering through an area with little edible food and limited amounts to drink, they needed mechanisms to conserve their nutrients, salt and fluid to maintain a healthy blood pressure. This would ensure a steady supply of glucose to their brains, which in turn prevented their minds from becoming clouded, feelings of disorientation, and unconsciousness.

Therefore the hunter-gatherers developed protective fat-storage mechanisms to guard them against the perils of an inconsistent supply of food and water. They feasted on anything that was available through either hunting or gathering. The storage mechanisms would eagerly mop up any over-indulgence and save it, to help them to cope with times of famine when food wasn't so readily available. In this way human beings' metabolism became geared to survive through both feast and famine.

Although ancient man's life was damned inconvenient, his body certainly complemented his lifestyle. Modern man's body has basically the same metabolic processes as our hunter-gatherer ancestors, but our lifestyle has changed dramatically. The only hunting or gathering we do today is to drive the car to the local supermarket, pick up a large supply of processed, packaged rubbish (disguised as food), place it in the boot and drive home, where we preserve it in the pantry or the fridge. Although this is quick and easy, it does not match our physiology and is a major contributor to our modern ills.

When we consider the necessities for human survival, what are we doing to attain them? Instead of seeking and satisfying these needs through normal, nature-based mechanisms, we have invented all kinds of artificial, synthetic substitutes. We tend to opt for the most convenient route. With careful planning, we can almost eradicate the need to expend any physical and mental energy at all. In the majority of cases this makes survival much easier, but I strongly believe that the convenient acquisition of our basic needs is killing us.

Life in the modern world appears to be squarely focused on the accumulation of wealth and material goods. We are also developing an extraordinary knowledge base that is allowing scientists, engineers and others to design all manner of items that are intended purely to make our lives more comfortable.

Although modern life has many advantages and although our bodies have been designed in an extraordinary manner, with significant reserves and safety mechanisms to ensure prolonged survival, we are pushing these mechanisms to the limit with our modern 'convenient' lifestyle. Our growing epidemics of obesity, diabetes and cancer, along with the ongoing carnage from cardiovascular disease, are testaments to this. As I have said, it is my firm belief that 'convenience is killing us', and we cannot rely upon the medical profession to solve these problems once they have occurred.

If you do not want convenience to be your killer, start thinking about how you can go back to a more natural style of living within the realm of our modern world. All the answers are in this book. Firstly, let's look at the advantages of our modern age.

ADVANTAGE 1: FOOD

In the Western world, time is a precious commodity. Our ancestors would spend hours catching, gathering and preparing food and then just as long consuming it. Now we have an increasing dependence on eating take-away, pre-packaged or microwaved foods, which reduces our need to spend time in preparation.

ADVANTAGE 2: SHELTER

When our Hunter-Gatherer friend returned home to his cave after a hard day in the jungle, he greeted his pre-historic wife and children, settled on his favourite piece of sand and turned on the 'idiot rock' to watch some futuristic TV show about a family known as the Flint-stones . . . Well, maybe it didn't go quite like that, but you get the picture (even though he didn't)! Life for our hunter-gatherer ancestors was simple and straightforward. There were no mortgages, stock exchanges, lawsuits or doctors' bills. Life was purely about surviving for as long and as well as you could, living in whatever shelter was available.

These days, it is the great 'modern dream' to own our home, which is usually equipped with every modern convenience, such as air conditioners, alarms, pools, entertainment systems and appliances, to minimise the need to spend time on life's menial tasks. These conveniences allow us to avoid the extremes of hot and cold endured for millennia by our ancestors. They give us additional comfort when we are sleeping, as our beds and mattresses are designed by chiropractors who, of all people, must know what constitutes a comfortable, back-friendly bed because they spend all day cracking the backs of people who have obviously never slept on a chiropractor-sanctioned bed!

ADVANTAGE 3: ENTERTAINMENT

Over the last ten years or so we have witnessed an explosion of push-button entertainment, such as free-to-air and pay television, computer games, DVDs and videos. Some pay television facilities offer hundreds of channels to cater for even the most bizarre tastes. The wonderful advantage here is that we no longer have to struggle with our own imaginations – it's all laid down for us. Scenarios are created to delight our senses without our ever having to leave the comfort of our lounge room, or use our mind.

ADVANTAGE 4: TRANSPORT

We live in a global world. Our transport has become so sophisticated that the need to use our legs to move is diminishing rapidly. Modern communications no longer require us to deliver messages in person. We can (and often do) send an email to the person in the next room.

ADVANTAGE 5: INFORMATION TECHNOLOGY

We are truly living in the information age. Since the introduction of the Internet, we can access information about any subject we like. There are multiple services available online, including banking, shopping, financial and health advice.

No doubt modern society has its advantages, and these have caused extraordinary improvements in our quality of life. But there are also disadvantages that arise in consequence of these modern conveniences.

DISADVANTAGE 1: TECHNOLOGY

The twentieth and twenty-first centuries have brought with them an extraordinary burgeoning of technology, which has had major consequences on society. One is that we have access to a vast array of food stuffs that do not need to be consumed immediately. For these foods to be preserved and packaged, it is necessary for synthetic chemicals to be added. The ready availability of these foods ensures that they are consumed on a regular basis.

Technology has guaranteed that our bodies are not only bombarded with subtle (and at times not so subtle) doses of synthetic chemicals in our food, but also that these are used to create our appliances, 'aids to daily living', clothing, and detergent to wash our clothes and ourselves.

Constant movement is a central aspect of normal metabolism, maintenance of a healthy cardiovascular system, muscle tone and lubrication of our joints. We have replaced this constant movement with (in those of us who bother to exercise) bursts of activity in between hours of sedentary behaviour. I am always amused by the person who is surprised that they are not losing weight despite their half an hour of exercise on three occasions per week, whilst the remainder of the time they are performing little or no movement whatsoever.

DISADVANTAGE 2: SYNTHETIC CHEMICALS

Modern synthetic chemicals contribute to our current health problems in four main areas, which are outlined below.

Synthetic chemicals and nutrition

'If you can kill it and eat it straightaway or grow it in your backyard then it's good for you.' This old-style, natural approach to nutrition has been lost. Modern foods are laced with synthetic fats (or 'trans fats'; see *The Cell Factor*), processed carbohydrates and numerous other addictives that allow food to sit in a container on a shelf for months.

SYNTHETIC CHEMICALS AND HYGIENE

In our modern world, being hygienic is equated with good health. Hygiene is a word often used by experts and authorities denoting goodness. Interestingly, however, excessive hygiene may also have its drawbacks. My grandfather used to say, 'If a child hasn't eaten the equivalent of a bucket of dirt by the age of five, it's not healthy'. Studies over the past ten years have shown a higher incidence of allergies and asthma in children brought up in a more hygienic environment. Children from lower socioeconomic groups and less hygienic conditions had higher rates of respiratory tract infections but fewer allergic conditions. These are not just the conditions that we would typically associate with allergies – asthma, hay fever and eczema; the main allergy to emerge over the past ten to 15 years is food allergy.

A study from the UK has shown that allergies to peanuts tripled between 1989 and 1996. Another study, from New York, showed that food allergies doubled between 1997 and 2002.

The initial theory regarding this marked rise in allergies was that it was due to the elimination of serious childhood infections through improved hygiene, immunisations and antibiotics, but there did not appear to be a logical link here. Recently, my grandfather's theory has been shown to 'have legs' – the rise in allergies is almost certainly due to lack of exposure to the harmless bugs that live in dirt and stimulate certain cells within the immune system, thereby blocking the allergens' assault. Our immune systems need to be challenged in the same way that our muscles need exercise. Since we have stopped children playing outside in parks, in the dirt, in the bush, and we live in a world where we are increasingly vigilant about the dangers posed by the outside world, our sterile environments and synthetic-based living quarters hold no place for the helpful bugs that are only found outdoors. Our children, although protected from the outside dangers, are facing a new threat, this time from within their own bodies.

Another problem with hygiene is the effect of all the synthetic chemicals we use to maintain it. We are being exposed all day, every day, to micro levels of synthetics, from the stuff we spray, rub and soak into our bodies to the cleaning materials for our clothes, linen, plates, houses and cars.

DEODORANT AND ALUMINIUM

There is no doubt that the most effective deodorant is one that contains aluminium, but there is an ongoing debate regarding its safety. Aluminium has been implicated as a factor in Alzheimer's disease and breast cancer. Using aluminium directly to the armpit area theoretically delivers high-concentration aluminium straight into the axillary lymph nodes, and possibly into the breasts. Recently, a study of breast cancer sufferers versus an age-matched control group showed no increased risk of breast cancer amongst the users of aluminium-based deodorants. Whilst this doesn't disprove the theory, it does cast doubt on it.

Lack of social contacts through non-use of an aluminium-based deodorant may make you so miserable that the loneliness and social isolation become a factor in the generation of your heart disease or cancer . . . you can't win sometimes.

Synthetic chemicals and air pollution

Our air, which once was pure, is now loaded with thousands of pollutants. Evidence is mounting to support the theory that air pollution is a factor in the rising rates of respiratory diseases, including cancers, in large cities. Studies show clearly that many modern diseases are more common in urban dwellers than in those living in rural areas. It is said that people living in the country live for seven years longer than city dwellers. (We urbanites would argue that it just feels like seven years!)

These days breathing outdoors in a large city is a health hazard in itself. With the ubiquitous burning of fossil-based fuels by industry and cars, we are daily being exposed to thousands of toxic chemicals by the simple act of breathing.

Many of us work and live in environments where the air is artificial. This is, of course, necessary to maintain a reasonable air temperature and avoid the pollutants from the outside environment.

During winter, many of us will come down with a cold or virus. It is my opinion that it is not bad to pick up these conditions occasionally as it gives the immune system a bit of a work-out. However, a recent study in the *Respiratory Care Journal* has suggested something that most of us have suspected for many years. Large inner-city office blocks (where more people are tending to work), which have a low supply of outdoor air, are more likely to harbour viruses in their air filters than better ventilated buildings. A common respiratory pathogen (or bug) known as a picornavirus was found in around 30 per cent of office building air-sampling filters.

Although our society dictates that concentrated activity in large office buildings is the most efficient way to organise modern corporate life, as usual, this artificial approach to living comes at a price. It seems that 'sick' buildings produce sick people.

Nicotine

Just when you thought medical science had completely understood the toxic effects of cigarette smoke, yet another surprising study has been released that links passive cigarette smoking and breast cancer. Strangely, there seems to be a much closer association between passive smoking and breast cancer than there is between active smoking and the disease.

On 9 March 2005, *USA Today* released a report from the Centre of Disease Control in the United States, which reviewed 1000 studies of the health effects of passive smoking. The researchers claimed that those exposed to passive smoking had a greater risk (90 per cent) of breast cancer than active smokers. They also believe that just over 73,000 people die in the United States each year as a direct consequence of passive smoking (not just from breast cancer). The study suggested that the more extensive and the earlier the exposure, especially if this was before puberty or a first pregnancy, the higher the risk became.

There is a link between breast cancer and high levels of oestrogen. It appears that the high levels of cancer-producing substances found in the bloodstream of active cigarette smokers blocks the oestrogen receptors in the breast. It is felt that this explains the lower risk of breast cancer seen in active smokers. Strangely, lower dose cancer-producing substances, such as cigarette smoke inhaled by passive smokers, appear to stimulate the same receptors and thus switch on the oestrogen receptors in the breast. This doesn't mean that smoking protects against cancer, as the rates of lung cancer in cigarette smokers far outweigh the rates of breast cancer in passive smokers.

A recently released study from Britain has followed cigarette smokers for 50 years. It reported that the earlier a person gives up smoking, the more benefits they gain. Despite this, even if someone stops smoking at the age of 60, they live for three years longer than someone who continues to smoke. If a person stops smoking at the age of 30, they live a staggering 10 years longer than an ongoing smoker. The study showed that two-thirds of smokers will die as a direct consequence of cigarettes.

Air pollutants

In the early 1970s, when I started medical school, my first after-hours job was working as a car park attendant. My boss had been working in the car park for the previous 30 years. He later died in his seventies, of severe Parkinson's disease.

In our increasingly synthetic world where we are exposed to a number of significant pollutants, it seems that chronic neurologic disorders, such as Parkinson's and Alzheimer's disease, are increasing markedly. A recent study from the UK has demonstrated that chronic exposure to environmental poisons such as pesticides, industrial effluents and car exhaust fumes is closely related to the incidence of brain disorders. There was a 300 per cent increase of these disorders in men and a 90 per cent increase in women between 1979 and 1997.

A study from France recently revealed that children living next to a petrol station or a mechanic's workshop had an eight-fold increase in risk of leukemia compared with children who did not live close to one of these.

DISADVANTAGE 3: IRRADIATION

A few years ago I was lecturing in Arizona, and friends suggested a trip to Sedona, which is famous for its alternative community and is said to be a place of intense natural energies. There are allegedly regions on this earth with concentrated, subtle energies (known by some as Vortices) that have magical healing properties. These hotly disputed energies form the basis of many ancient religions and modern 'energy medicine'. I visited the community in Sedona, purchased a Vortex map and stood (with a few other hopeful travellers) in the areas marked on the map. I felt nothing.

I may have been having a bad-Vortex day, or the Vortex concept may have no validity whatsoever. Either way, no-one disputes the existence of energy in its more well documented forms.

Extremely low frequencies of electromagnetic energy (from 25 to 300 hertz (Hz)) have not been found to be dangerous. The earth's magnetic field delivers energy at around 10 Hz, and the human pineal gland, which is found in the brain and is considered to be an important controlling factor on biologic processes, resonates at around 8 Hz.

Not all electromagnetic fields are harmful. But there are some that may be, and that might be easily overlooked.

Irradiation and household appliances

It is felt by some authorities that a particularly dangerous form of electromagnetic field is the 'out of sight' electrical wiring in houses. Although these only give out low frequencies (around 50 Hz), they deliver a continuous signal and, if you are in one place for an extended period (for example, for approximately eight hours at night), any repeated exposure may have subtle long-term effects, which are difficult to quantify.

Our bedrooms may be intense electromagnetic fields. Many people have televisions in their bedroom, and hold computers on their lap as they type in bed, checking the time on the bedside digital clock whilst warming their body with the electric blanket. Digital alarm clocks are necessary for many of us, but it might be wise to position them as far away from the bed as possible.

MICROWAVES AND RADIATION

The microwave oven is a common item in most kitchens. A recent segment on the Australian television program *Today Tonight* presented a report on microwaving food, suggesting that it might cause low-level radiation. The report went on to suggest that childhood leukemia is increased with long-term exposure to electromagnetic radiation, and suggested a vague connection between this radiation and exposure to microwaves.

The leading Australian nutritionist Dr Rosemary Stanton, however, disputes these findings. She suggests that most of the microwave scare comes from a particular Swiss chemist, Hans Hertel, whom, she claims, has used some spurious science to denigrate the benefits of microwave cooking. She does admit that steaming is the best way of cooking vegetables, as it retains more vitamins and minerals, but she states that most of the studies claiming a marked reduction in vitamin, mineral and other phyto-chemical content from microwaving found that this was purely because the foods were over-cooked or not cooked at the correct temperature. (Excessively microwaving your vegetables destroys 90 per cent of the phyto-chemicals – vitamins, minerals, trace chemicals – essential for good health.)

IRRADIATION AND CHILDREN

A recent study in *USA Today* reported that the amount of time that the eight- to 18-year-old age group spends using electronic devices per day is as follows:

Activity	Approximate time spent per day
Watching television	4 hours
Listening to music	1 hour 45 minutes
Using a computer	1 hour
Playing video games	50 minutes
Watching movies	25 minutes

This is an extraordinary amount of time to be exposed to electronics. I see five major issues: possible electromagnetic radiation, lack of physical activity, lack of social interaction, children's imaginations being fed for them by other media rather than using their own brain, and violence experienced through television and video games.

Irradiation and sunlight

With the increase in global warming and the expanding hole in the ozone layer, we are being exposed to harmful ultraviolet rays. In Australia especially, our rates of skin cancer are going through the roof. However, the main source of vitamin D for humans is sunlight, and because we are trying to avoid excessive sun exposure, our doses of this vitamin are decreasing. The resulting vitamin D deficiency can lead to osteoporosis, and over the last 20 to 30 years, the skin cancer epidemic has been rivalled by this condition.

At a recent paediatric bone symposium held in Sydney, a study reported that one in eight fair-skinned women were deficient in vitamin D. This was compared to one in five dark-skinned women and three out of four women who wore veils. The findings led the researchers to suggest that women should be having a dose of sunlight every day, especially during times of high vitamin D and calcium demand, such as pregnancy. A proposal of ten minutes' sunshine per day was made, which will help to alleviate vitamin D deficiency and its resulting health problems.

Irradiation and mobile phones

Many people have ongoing concerns about the risk of mobile phone use. Two recent studies, published in the *American Journal of Epidemiology* and *Epidemiology*, have added to the confusion. The first study, from Denmark, compared over 100 cases of mobile users with just over 200 matched controls and found no difference between mobile phone use and non-use and the risk of an acoustic neuroma, which is a benign tumour of the nerve to the inner ear.

Interestingly, however, the second study, from Sweden, compared around 150 cases of acoustic neuroma with 600 controls, and showed that after ten years or more of mobile phone use, the risk of acoustic neuroma was twice as large in mobile phone users than in non-users. When they looked at the risk of tumours on the same side of the head that the phone was used, the risk was four times greater.

It would be interesting to find out who sponsored these particular trials because, in my experience, most negative results in mobile phones trials (that is, those that show that mobile phones are harmless) are sponsored by telecommunication companies, as opposed to the trials that show harmful effects of mobile phone use, which are usually independent.

When we examine most modern illnesses, the concept of risk factors comes into play. A risk factor increases your risk of disease but its presence does not mean you will definitely contract the disease. It may be that mobile phones increase the risk of brain tumours in susceptible people (who have other factors – maybe genetic – that predispose them to the disease).

It is my opinion that mobile phones have not been proven safe in the long term and, although they are necessary in our society, their use should be restricted.

Although there are many advantages to living in our modern world, we are being exposed more and more to the disadvantages. We choose to live in this society, but I believe it is important that we try to minimise our exposure to its chemical and environmental hazards. Later chapters will outline principles for doing this.

CHAPTER 2

Free radicals

I believe that modern living is an internal battle to stay healthy, keep fit, cope with stress, maintain a normal weight, avoid disease and, ultimately, achieve longevity. With all battles, there are good guys and bad guys. The bad guys for humans are free radicals: highly reactive chemicals which distort, damage or destroy normal chemicals and tissues in the body that are necessary for healthy functioning.

When we introduce any synthetic chemical or any type of stress to our body, high levels of oxygen and energy are needed to deal with it. Any excessive use of oxygen produces free radicals. So, huge quantities of free radicals are generated, because in our modern Western world we are in constant contact with a vast array of synthetic chemicals and stresses.

Free radicals lack an electron (a negatively charged ion within the nucleus of an atom) and are therefore unstable. They attempt to achieve stability by stealing electrons from body tissues. This process is known as oxidation, and it causes the tissues from which the electrons are removed to become unstable, threatening their health.

To return to the battle analogy, I see the body as an invaded country. The free radicals are trying to attack it, to steal its electrons. For protection, the country needs an army and a robust defence system. These two lines of defence are provided by antioxidants (the army) and cell membranes (the defence).

ANTIOXIDANTS

Antioxidants are molecules found in many foods and in the body, and they sacrifice themselves by giving up their electrons to free radicals, to prevent the body's tissues from being attacked.

Free radicals don't particularly care where they obtain their electrons from, so they will accept the antioxidant electrons. For this to happen, the antioxidants need to be in the body at the time of attack. In a 'natural' environment, the combination of healthy food consumed in appropriate quantities and the body's own internal antioxidant system would be enough to neutralise the free radicals produced by day-to-day living. However, with modern Western society's excessive production of free radicals, it is difficult to obtain the necessary amount of antioxidants. One of the most important principles of balance between free radicals and antioxidants is the daily consumption of large doses of antioxidants in all their available forms. The four main natural sources of antioxidants are listed below.

ANTIOXIDANT 1: FRUITS AND VEGETABLES

I suggest eating two or three pieces of fruit and between three and five servings of vegetables per day. (A serving is, on average, half a standard cup.) People consuming this amount will have the lowest rate of heart disease and cancer in their community.

When we consider antioxidants, we usually think of vitamin E, vitamin C and betacarotene, which can be viewed as the 'work horses' of the group. However, there are hundreds of antioxidants in all fruits and vegetables, which are known collectively as phyto-chemicals (from the Greek, *phyto*, meaning plant).

Blueberries and strawberries

Of all the fruits, these two berries have the highest amounts of antioxidants. One serving of blueberries is around a quarter of a standard cup; one serving of strawberries is three or four average-size fruits.

Seeds

This is a part of fruit or vegetables that we usually discard, but if the seeds can be eaten, I advise doing so. Grape seeds, for example, contain powerful antioxidants, and in laboratory experiments they have been found to be much more potent than vitamin E or vitamin C. Seeds should not be swallowed whole, as their protective hard coating will prevent digestion. Chew them before swallowing, and this will enable the antioxidants to enter the body's system.

Green vegetables

Recently, scientists in Britain have found a chemical known as sinigrin, a chemical compound from the brassica family of vegetables, which includes broccoli, spinach, cabbage, cauliflower and brussels sprouts. Interestingly, sinigrin is involved in the processing of a chemical known as AITC (allyl-isothiocyanate), which is a form of cyanide. When AITC is released into a cancer cell, it stops it from dividing (the way in which cancer spreads). Sinigrin and its active chemical, AITC, does not occur naturally in the body and must be obtained from healthy foods.

Antioxidant 2: extra virgin olive oil

Extra virgin olive oil has large amounts of antioxidants as well as good monounsaturated fats. It is olive oil in its most natural form (if the oil is processed further, the number of antioxidants it contains is reduced). Cook with it, put it on salads and dip wholegrain bread in it!

Antioxidant 3: tea

Most people are aware of the longevity of people from Japan. One of the suggested reasons for this is the nation's partiality to green tea. This type of tea has the highest concentration of antioxidants of all the varieties. The region where green tea is produced has the lowest rates of heart disease and cancer in all of Japan.

Standard black tea (with or without milk) has plenty of antioxidants, though not as many as the green variety. It is estimated that around 30 per cent of antioxidant intake in Australia comes from the regular ingestion of tea.

HERBAL TEAS

These have recently become popular in the West. Most contain few or no antioxidants, but are beneficial in other areas. Peppermint tea, for example, is helpful for people with digestive problems, especially irritable bowel syndrome sufferers, and camomile tea has relaxant properties, so may be of some use in relieving stress.

ANTIOXIDANT 4: RED WINE

In my opinion, a daily low dose of red wine is beneficial to the health. Over the past 20 years, medical researchers in Boston have been assessing groups of men and women, monitoring aspects of their health and determining which factors prevent or induce disease. The male study recently reported that those men who ingested one to two small glasses of red wine per day had 80 per cent fewer sudden cardiac deaths and 50 per cent less heart disease and cancer compared with those who drank no red wine. The research also showed that moderate red wine consumption had a protective effect on kidney function.

Those men who consumed around two standard drinks (125ml of wine per drink) a day had a 30 per cent lower risk of kidney damage than those who drank no alcohol.

Vitamin supplements

As I mentioned at the start of the chapter, if we lived in a 'natural' world, where we were only exposed to natural chemicals and foods, we would achieve a healthy balance between free radicals and antioxidants.

In our modern Western world of excessive synthetic chemicals and chronic stress, we have an imbalance in favour of free radicals and, judging from the high occurrence of the free radical-based diseases (heart disease, cancer, chronic neurologic and inflammatory conditions) that make up the vast majority of modern illnesses, we cannot be receiving enough antioxidants from a healthy diet alone.

It seems to me that the only way to neutralise these excessive doses of free radicals is with supplemental antioxidants. This is a controversial opinion that most health care professionals disagree with, as they believe that supplements are merely an unbeneficial expense. Nevertheless, I am a strong believer in the regular ingestion of appropriate doses of natural supplementation.

An antioxidant dose of vitamin C is the equivalent of ten oranges. Although I would support someone consuming this number of oranges, I don't know too many people who could do so each day! To ingest the required daily antioxidant dose of vitamin E would mean eating two kilograms of margarine. I certainly would not recommend or endorse anyone doing this. As I see it, the only way to take in adequate doses of antioxidants is to consume as many of the foods mentioned above as regularly as possible, and to also ingest high-quality natural supplements.

Although in almost all occasions vitamins and other natural treatments have minimal side effects or long-term problems, it is my firm belief that a program of supplements should be supervised by a health professional.

CELL MEMBRANES

The second line of defence against free radical attack is formed by our cell membranes, which cover every cell in the body, and could be seen as individual castles. These membranes are 75 per cent fat. Without a good supply of healthy fat, they become leaky and unhealthy.

Cell membranes help to determine metabolism rate. Large animals like whales and elephants, with slow metabolisms, have thick, water-tight cell membranes that contain saturated fatty acids. Small animals such as mice or humming birds, with quick metabolisms, have thin, runny, leaky membranes containing polyunsaturated fats as their main bulk.

Polyunsaturated fats are vital for the rapid transfer of information. Therefore, for animals who rely on quick reactions for survival (usually small animals), polyunsaturated fats in the cells of the nervous system are imperative. If the brain does not have an adequate supply of polyunsaturated fat, it doesn't work as well. These animals also use lots of energy and oxygen, which leads to the production of large numbers of free radicals.

In contrast, large animals, with high levels of saturated fats in their brains, are slow-witted and half blind, but produce fewer free radicals.

This can help to explain why large animals tend to have much greater life spans than those that are small: free radical production is much lower in larger animals, so they are exposed to less risk of disease, and their aging process is slower.

Over the past 50 years, saturated fats have been implicated as the major reason for high cholesterol, heart disease and obesity. I believe that the evidence for this is quite weak. Saturated fat comes mainly from sources such as animal fats and dairy products, and from isolated food stuffs like coconut oil and cashew nuts. The food industry, which makes most money from processed, packaged foods with a long shelf-life, is happy for these natural food sources to be unpopular. However, the body needs a reasonable amount of saturated fat and cholesterol for cell membrane stability. It also needs the correct blend of healthy polyunsaturated fats.

In my opinion, the chemically altered, synthetically processed polyunsaturated fats (or trans fats) in packaged foods contribute to modern disease more than saturated fat. Although saturated fat slows down the metabolism and makes cell membranes more sticky and water-tight (which may reduce the normal flow of nutrients into the cell and therefore should not be consumed in excess), trans fats, even in low doses, should be avoided more stringently. As little as a two per cent increase in trans fat consumption can lead to up to a 90 per cent increase in risk of a heart attack. (For more information on trans fats, there is extensive coverage in my book *The Cell Factor*.)

Omega 3

Omega 3 is a form of polyunsaturated fat found in fish, flaxseed oil, egg white and various nuts. It plays a vital role in keeping the body healthy. All cell membranes need fat, and will take any fat that is around at the time. A diet high in Omega 3 ensures that the membranes stay healthy, allowing a normal exchange of nutrients and other chemicals in and out of the cells. Some of its other benefits are listed below.

Omega 3 helps to lower blood fat levels

This means that the fats in the blood stream are less likely to contain the highly toxic LDL cholesterol, which free radicals find easy to oxidise. Omega 3 also tends to reduce levels of lipoprotein (a) (see Chapter 3).

Omega 3 acts as a blood thinner

The thinner your blood, the less likely it is to clot, meaning that if an artery in the heart ruptures (as a consequence of atherosclerosis, in which the arteries become clogged by fatty substances), it is less likely that a clot will form, block the artery and cause a heart attack.

Omega 3 is an anti-inflammatory

There is a group of important chemicals known as eicosanoids. These ecosanoids work at the cellular level and determine the body's inflammatory response. Omega 3s generate beneficial eicosanoids that are anti-inflammatory and thus reduce the risk for all manner of cardiovascular events such as heart attack, angina, stroke and sudden cardiac death.

Omega 3 helps the heart to function normally

The heart's electrical system is made from a series of natural wires, and Omega 3 ensures that these wires are bathed in healthy fats. Anyone consuming a diet high in Omega 3 not only has a reduced heart attack rate, but also has a greater reduction in heart rhythm disorders (arrhythmia) and sudden cardiac death.

CASE STUDY: OMEGA 3 AND HEART FUNCTION

A man in his sixties complained of palpitations (irregular heart beats). After investigations with a 24-hour heart monitor, which showed frequent but benign ectopic (abnormal) heart beats, I prescribed 4 grams of fish oil per day.

His condition was reviewed one month later, and he stated that his palpitations had stopped. As a bonus, his golf swing had improved, because the anti-inflammatory properties of the oil had increased mobility in his shoulder!

As we have seen, it is not possible to ward off free radical attacks completely with antioxidants derived from a healthy diet, but there is no doubt that consuming a diet high in antioxidant-based foods reduces the risk of heart disease, diabetes and cancer.

It is important to understand that modern Western diseases are primarily caused by free radical attack. When our bodies encounter modern society (with its excess of synthetic chemicals and stress), our body tissues are invaded, oxidised and subsequently damaged by free radicals, which leaves them vulnerable to disease. It is too simplistic to see heart disease as a condition of too much fat in the arteries. This might be the final result, but the disease began with free radicals assaulting the entire vascular system. The following chapter considers two reasons for our bodies being insufficiently defended against modern levels of free radical attack.

CHAPTER 3

Evolutionary problems

Our modern world appears to be coming up with ways to induce disease in its inhabitants. Some of these diseases are related to the increasing doses of synthetic chemicals to which we are exposed, whilst others are associated with our sedentary lifestyles. With our inactive forms of entertainment, not to mention the extraordinary advances in technology allowing most tasks to be performed at the touch of a button, our lack of movement is causing significant health issues. 'Diabesity', the combination of weight gain and late-onset diabetes, is the most significant issue related to a sedentary lifestyle. The condition has led to an extraordinary increase in cardiovascular disease.

These days, the average male can hope to survive to his late seventies, and the average female to her early eighties (although the most recent mortality statistics show that there has actually been a drop in our longevity rates). Around 45 per cent of people in modern Western society will die from some form of cardiovascular disease, whilst around 30 per cent will die from cancer.

As we saw in Chapter 1, our hunter-gatherer ancestors evolved survival mechanisms that improved their chances of good health and longevity. These mechanisms are still part of modern humans' physiology, but instead of aiding our survival, they do just the opposite, creating conditions in the body that increase the risk of disease. We will consider two of these risks to survival in this chapter.

SURVIVAL RISK 1: INSULIN RESISTANCE

On most of the cells in our bodies, including those in our muscles and major organs, are 'doorways' known as energy receptors. These control the flow of fuel (in the form of glucose or fat) into the cell, allowing the appropriate regulation of energy flow and ensuring that the cells receive an even supply – neither more nor less than is required for them to function normally. The cells of the brain and those concerned with fat do not have these energy receptors, which enables fuel to flow freely into them.

When we consume food that contains fats or sugars, the pancreas releases insulin, a hormone, into the blood. Insulin is the 'doorman' that makes the energy receptors in the cells open, enabling the regulated flow of nutrients.

If an individual is insulin resistant, the receptor doesn't open properly, thus reducing the normal flow of fuel (glucose or fat) into the cell. The only mechanism the body has for coping with this is to produce more insulin, thus forcing the receptor to open to allow the fuel to enter the cell.

The resulting high levels of insulin (through mechanisms not as yet specifically determined) raise the blood pressure and alter the cholesterol profile. High levels of insulin also lay down visceral fat, thus the epidemic of abdominal obesity.

In an individual who is not insulin resistant, glucose (either in the diet or made primarily in the liver) and, to a lesser extent, fat, stimulates an appropriate balanced amount of insulin, ensuring the necessary amount of fuel in the cell.

WHY WAS INSULIN RESISTANCE BENEFICIAL FOR OUR ANCESTORS?

We know that the hunter-gatherers' entire lives were based around feast and famine. When food was available, the reduced entry of fuel into the insulin resistant cells ran a slightly higher blood sugar level, keeping the brain supplied with a healthy dose of fuel and, along with sugar, acting as a substrate for fat production by the fat cells.

This was a most effective survival mechanism for the hunter-gatherers.

Why is insulin resistance unbeneficial for modern Western humans?

Food is readily available and we eat when we are hungry. An over-abundance of regular food supplies means that modern insulin resistant humans overstock their fat stores and have much higher blood sugar levels than are necessary for quality survival; they also overwork their pancreas, creating unhealthily high insulin levels.

Insulin resistance occurs in around 30 per cent of Caucasians, 50 to 60 per cent of Asians and almost 100 per cent of people with dark skin. It might have been an aid to survival for hunter-gatherers but, if not managed properly, will significantly threaten existence in the modern world.

Signs of insulin resistance

There are five common indicators of insulin resistance in modern humans:

Sign 1: central (abdominal) obesity

This is the hallmark of insulin resistance and is a strong indication of fat accumulating around the more important organs and the arteries.

A simple way to discover if you have central obesity is to measure the circumference of your waist. In males, a circumference of over 100 centimetres means that you are centrally obese; in women, obesity is confirmed by a measurement of over 89 centimetres. Monitoring central obesity using a tape measure, your belt size or how well you can see your feet when standing up are excellent methods of determining if you might be storing unhealthy levels of fat.

Sign 2: cholesterol abnormalities

Cholesterol is a vital part of our body. Without cholesterol in our cell walls or acting as the basic building block for many of our hormones we would perish. However, abnormal cholesterol levels in the blood can indicate insulin resistance.

People living in hunter-gatherer communities that exist today have cholesterol levels below 3 millimoles per litre, compared with the average 4–5.5 level for modern Western humans. As hunter-gatherer communities eat no processed food and consume fewer daily calories than people in the West, their metabolisms cannot generate cholesterol above this level. We can assume that our hunter-gatherer ancestors had similar cholesterol levels.

CHOLESTEROL MISCONCEPTIONS

Over the past 20 to 30 years, society has become cholesterol obsessed. These are two common misconceptions about cholesterol:

- Cholesterol is often said to be the cause of fat deposits in the arteries, but it is actually more a marker for our degree of nutrition. Progressive build-up of fat in the arteries is a condition called atherosclerosis, which can lead to heart attack, stroke and sudden death. If you are over-nourished, you will deposit fat in your arteries and if you are under-nourished, you will not.

- Cholesterol is regularly associated with cardiovascular disease, but it is wrong to suggest a direct link between the two; high cholesterol levels do not always mean that a cardiovascular problem will develop. Equally, having normal cholesterol levels does not necessarily protect a person against the disease. Around 30 to 40 per cent of heart attack sufferers have totally normal cholesterol levels.

Sign 3: hypertension

Hypertension, or high blood pressure, is a common feature of insulin resistance. Many researchers believe that the insulin resistant gene raises blood pressure.

Sign 4: diabetes

Insulin resistance is the basic cause for late-onset diabetes. (Insulin-dependent diabetes is a totally different disease, usually present in childhood, with insulin treatment being the main therapy.)

Although an individual is insulin resistant from birth, they may never become a diabetic. However, diabetes occurs when the pancreas, which has been overworked from birth to cope with the insulin resistance, eventually cannot keep up with the insulin demand, and the blood sugar level starts to rise. This results in the excess sugar binding to various proteins in the blood, tissues and cells, creating toxic chemicals that promote the growth of fatty plaques (the portions of the blood vessel walls where fat accumulates) and clog the small blood vessels to the eyes, kidneys and nerves, leading to accelerated atherosclerosis, diabetic eye disease, and diabetic kidney and nerve damage.

Sign 5: cardiovascular disease

Insulin resistance markedly increases the risk of this disease.

CASE STUDY: INSULIN RESISTANCE

Eddie was a 47-year-old male referred to me because of non-specific chest pain occurring beneath his left breast and lasting for around a minute at a time. His pain was not related to exertion and was intermittent. He suffered no other symptoms apart from some mild shortness of breath, as he was unfit.

Eddie had a round face, was of average height, had thick hands and fingers, and suffered from central obesity. He craved sweets and biscuits, and preferred warm weather. He had been thin in his teens, but his love of sweets, cola-based drinks, and biscuits had led to progressive weight gain over 25 years. His weight was a major concern for the future. However, after commencing a high-protein, high-fat diet, Eddie had lost considerable weight.

Eddie had no previous history of cardiac problems. Both parents had developed late-onset diabetes, but there was no family history of heart disease. Eddie was a non-smoker and was not diabetic. Test results showed that he had higher than average cholesterol levels and slightly raised blood pressure.

Eddie's chest pain was musculo-skeletal in origin and related to his years of heavy lifting in the building trade. Although I could reassure him regarding his pain, he had numerous other potential health issues that needed addressing.

The simplest explanation for Eddie's other health problems related to the various effects of dieting in different people. The high-protein, high-fat diet that Eddie had used burns fat rapidly (especially with his particular body type – see Part 3). This leads to a marked increase in fat entering the circulation, which the liver then tries to eliminate. The extra fat burden on Eddie's system was reflected in his liver function tests; insulin resistance sufferers commonly have a condition known as a fatty liver.

Unfortunately, the body takes up to six months to restore itself to some type of sensible balance after this type of diet. One of Eddie's tests showed an increase in cholesterol and triglycerides (fats), which was a reflection of the fat deposited in the circulation due to the diet. With time and ongoing weight loss Eddie's cholesterol and triglyceride levels would return to more normal amounts.

SURVIVAL RISK 2: LIPOPROTEIN (a)

Lipoprotein (a) is a type of fat found in the body, which consists of a 'bad' cholesterol molecule (LDL) and a protein tail (apoprotein (a)). For a more detailed explanation of lipoprotein (a), see *The Cell Factor*.

Why was lipoprotein (a) beneficial for our ancestors?

A theory proposed by scientists Linus Pauling and Matthias Rath suggests that lipoprotein (a) was an evolutionary response to vitamin C deficiency.

Vitamin C is an important component of collagen (a structural protein). Human beings are one of a small number of mammals that do not produce the vitamin naturally within the body, and so need to access it from food. If a human's diet is deficient in the vitamin, they can develop scurvy, a disease characterised by a weakening of blood vessels due to the breakdown of collagen. People suffering from scurvy develop holes in their blood vessel walls, which can result in death.

Ancient humans had to evolve a mechanism for mending these holes during times of famine, and subsequent vitamin C deficiency, in order to survive. According to Pauling and Rath's theory, lipoprotein (a) evolved to act as a plug in the wall of blood vessels by supplying an extra dose of fat and by thickening the blood around the site of the hole.

Why is lipoprotein (a) unbeneficial for modern Western humans?

Our society has far more access to vitamin C-rich food, and few people in the West suffer from scurvy; therefore, lipoprotein (a) is not needed by modern humans. However, for people with high levels of lipoprotein (a) in their blood, it continues to deposit fat in artery walls and to thicken the blood. These two occurrences are best avoided in our modern world, as large amounts of fat and thick blood can lead to various aforementioned diseases.

HEALTH RISKS OF HIGH LIPOPROTEIN (a) LEVELS

Lipoprotein (a) is a purely genetic chemical. A person can be as healthy as possible in their lifestyle, but if their lipoprotein (a) is elevated, the risk of a heart attack or a related event is 70 per cent higher than that of a person with normal levels. The only way of knowing that your lipoprotein (a) is elevated is to have a specific blood test. An abnormally high Lp(a) occurs in 20 per cent of the general population.

There are two types of nutrients essential for normal body metabolism: macro-nutrients (fat, carbohydrates, or sugars, and protein) and micro-nutrients (vitamins, minerals and trace metals). For hunter-gatherers, being insulin resistant affected their macro-nutrient metabolism under feast and famine conditions. Having high lipoprotein (a) levels influenced the hunter-gatherers' micro-nutrient metabolism, protecting them against vitamin C deficiency.

In the modern Western world, with our lack of famine and increasingly sedentary lifestyles, the beneficial fat storage mechanisms (present in the hunter-gatherer) contribute to the modern plague of obesity, diabetes and cardiovascular diseases.

CHAPTER 4

Treating modern disease

One of the consistent aspects of medical science is that it is inconsistent. Every week, month, year and decade, the trends in disease prevention and therapy change.

If we had only one treatment for each condition, it would show that it worked. When there are a multitude of treatments that claim effectiveness, we can conclude that no one treatment is all that successful, or that the groups of people studied are responding differently to the various therapies. Therefore, if there appears to be a degree of confusion in the messages released to the public, that's because there is! There is certainly no consensus in medicine, and there will always be mixed messages, no matter how much 'evidence' is released.

As a medical professional, I am open to all aspects of medicine, including those that are integrative or complementary, and this has sometimes led people to form the wrong impression of my attitude to orthodox medicine. I have (mistakenly) developed a reputation as a cardiologist who can treat cardiac conditions without the use of orthodox treatments in the shape of drugs and surgery.

Two very interesting cases illustrate the point that the most sensible approach to treating disease is with a combination of both orthodox and complementary techniques.

CASE STUDY 1: CARDIOMYOPATHY AND STROKE

I recently gave a lecture to a company about the benefits of combining a healthy lifestyle with high-quality natural supplements. Soon after, a man in his sixties made an appointment to see me, to have his heart condition assessed. After hearing my lecture and misinterpreting my comments, he had decided to cease all of his medications, lead a healthy lifestyle and take supplements.

The man's case was fascinating. At the age of 34 he had been involved in a major car accident in which he suffered significant chest injuries. Whilst recovering in hospital, his pulse rate dropped intermittently to around 30 beats per minute. Within two years of the accident he required the insertion of a permanent pacemaker. He had remained well after this except that in the previous ten years he had noticed progressive shortness of breath. An echocardiogram (ultrasound of the heart) revealed a condition known as dilated cardiomyopathy (where the heart muscle swells with a marked reduction in its pumping ability). He had also suffered recurrent small strokes over the past few years.

The man had been on standard medical therapy (which included multiple drugs to treat his cardiomyopathy, and Warfarin to thin his blood and prevent any further strokes), but told me that since stopping all his treatment he had felt much better. He was surprised and disappointed when I expressed my disapproval of his course of action; he had thought that I would endorse his stopping the pills. Despite feeling much improved in the short term (as it is quite common for multiple medications to have side effects), ceasing medications without medical supervision (especially with a serious, chronic heart condition) was a dangerous and irresponsible step. The man's long-term cardiologist had provided him with expert and appropriate care.

I suggested that the man re-start his medication, along with improving his diet and exercise and making use of a tailored supplement program.

CASE STUDY 2: ATHEROSCLEROSIS

A 36-year-old man attended my clinic for a CT scan of his coronary arteries. (A CT scan is a non-invasive method of determining the amount of fat and calcium in the arteries, which are markers for atherosclerosis.) The scan showed a build-up of coronary calcium. After further testing, he was shown to have a significant elevation in his lipoprotein (a) levels. His father had suffered a heart attack and underwent coronary artery bypass grafting in his forties.

I suggested lifestyle modification, aspirin, cholesterol-lowering therapy and a supplement program. The man elected to follow the lifestyle and supplement programs but refused to take any other pills.

He returned to see me five years later, as he had been suffering from increasing chest pains. Tests had confirmed serious blockages in his coronary arteries. He had been referred to a cardiac surgeon, who thought that coronary artery bypass grafting was necessary and urgent. The man was unhappy with this suggestion and thought I might weave some magic without drugs or surgery. I confirmed the surgeon's opinions but the man had already made up his mind and refused to undergo an operation. However, after further chest pain there was no longer any choice, and the surgery was performed successfully.

Afterwards, with a combination of orthodox medicine and a complementary program, the man made good progress.

MANAGING SYMPTOMS

One of the major aspects of treating chronic medical problems is management of the symptoms. Unfortunately, it is a common misconception that the severity of symptoms indicates the severity of the underlying disease. I have seen many patients who wrongly felt that their condition was mild since they had either minimal or no symptoms. Symptoms should never be used by the sufferer as a signal of whether they do or don't have a problem.

Symptoms are 'tickets into the system', and are very useful for monitoring the individual's progress throughout a disease. Each person's case has to be judged individually; one size does not fit all, and it is dangerous to listen to your next-door neighbour! Any new symptoms should be assessed by a medical professional.

So many people ignore symptoms to their peril. I once saw a middle-aged male who had suffered from bleeding from the rectum for six months. He had wrongly diagnosed his condition as haemorrhoids, only to become extremely ill with bowel cancer.

Too many people are taken to the morgue with antacid tablets in their top pockets, having misdiagnosed their heart condition as indigestion.

PREVENTION

Why don't we put a stronger emphasis on prevention of disease during our lives? Probably because that's how we are built: nature will usually follow the line of least resistance – the simplest, easiest path. But the most successful human beings (in all aspects of life) are the planners, the goal-setters, the people who are disciplined enough to put in hard work. The most successful businesses are those where the people at the top are working 'on the business, not in the business'. Equally, the most successful human beings are those who are working on their lives, not in their lives. By this, I mean rather than spending the majority of the time dealing with life's urgent or, at times, menial issues, focus your efforts on improving and maintaining balance in all areas of your existence.

But cultivating discipline is not easy. We tend to deal with the urgent, pressing matters and leave the rest. We create living patterns that are hard to break and in the majority of cases those habits are contributing to our modern health problems. They include 'quick and easy' meals (whether microwaved at home or purchased at a take-away outlet); increasing dependency on forms of transport other than our legs; the overwhelming amount of time we spend travelling, working and climbing to the top; and the need for man-made solutions to our health problems.

Not only are we treating our bodies and minds wrongly, we are also being given the wrong messages by the medical and allied professions about how to be healthy. We are too quick to search for strong pharmaceutical agents to lower our cholesterol and blood pressure or to relieve our osteoporosis and joint pain, followed by surgery when the drugs are no longer effective.

Every time someone swallows a cholesterol pill, a blood pressure pill or an aspirin, they hope to prevent a heart problem, stroke or some other cardiovascular condition. But is there good evidence for these agents playing a preventative role?

Statin drugs and the Polypill

These medications in many cases reduce the risk of heart attack or stroke. All too frequently these days, a person will see their doctor, their only problem being elevated cholesterol, having no prior history of heart disease or other cardiac risk factors, and the doctor's immediate reaction is to reach for the script pad and prescribe a statin drug.

The reason for this seems straightforward to me, and is also disturbing: it's the easiest thing to do! It saves the doctor time that would be taken discussing diets, exercise, smoking and stress management which, if done properly, can take hours compared to the 30 seconds that it takes to write a prescription.

However, not all the blame lies with the doctor. There is also the matter of personal responsibility. It's much easier for the patient to swallow a pill than to make the necessary lifestyle changes that can make a significant impact on their health. This demonstrates another erosion of our own responsibility towards our bodies. It brings me back to one of the major themes of this book: convenience is killing us. If we believe a pill will reduce our risk of heart disease or stroke by a dramatic amount, there is then the subliminal message that we don't need to focus on lifestyle issues because the pill will do that for us.

Of course, there will be numerous occasions when lifestyle change alone is not enough. The judicious use of appropriate drug therapy is an important part of any cardiovascular preventative or therapeutic strategy, but it should never be the first line of attack.

Statin drugs do work, but only partially. Taken alone (without lifestyle interventions) in a standard dose, at best we can expect around a 30 per cent slowing of the disease process. In effect, this means that instead of having your heart attack in three years, you will have it in five.

These drugs also cause unwanted side effects, many of which may mimic the changes seen in the body with aging. Muscle pain and weakness, which appear gradually with the drugs over months, are often ascribed to arthritis and other age-related ailments.

There have been recent suggestions to create a Polypill which could contain a full dose statin drug, three half-dose blood pressure pills, low-dose aspirin and folic acid. The three blood pressure drugs (which include an ACE inhibitor, a beta-blocker and a calcium channel blocker) may cause a cough, shortness of breath and a myriad of other minor symptoms. The universal symptom of powerful pharmaceutical drugs, of course, is fatigue.

With only 45 per cent of people dying from cardiovascular disease, if we suggest everyone over the age of 55 takes a Polypill (as some medical professionals have done), then the majority of people taking it will be doing so unnecessarily. We are exposed to enough chemicals in this modern world without swallowing extra tablets on the premise that they may do some good.

It is likely that statin drugs and the Polypill will soon be available over the counter in Britain. I am horrified that powerful pharmaceutical preparations such as these might be made freely available to the public without close medical supervision. This is reducing them to the level of vitamin supplements. Even though we have the Internet for all kinds of DIY advice, I believe there is still an important place for professionals to supervise us with our health.

In my opinion, if someone is thought to be at high risk of heart attack or stroke, the combination of lifestyle change and appropriate medical treatment is the best approach to reversing the disease.

Aspirin

I am often asked whether people should take aspirin once they reach a certain age. Over the years there have been many opinions in medical circles about a daily dose of aspirin.

Studies in the late 1980s and early 1990s showed that taking one aspirin every day reduced the risk of heart attack by around 25 per cent. However, many of the studies were performed on people already at high risk of heart disease.

Around a third of the population have 'thick' blood that clots easily, with a minority of them suffering from serious clotting disorders. Another third have 'thin' blood that does not clot easily, with a small minority suffering from bleeding disorders such as haemophilia. The following case studies illustrate how aspirin can affect people with these different types of blood.

CASE STUDY 1: ASPIRIN AND THICK BLOOD

A very fit 40-year-old male paramedic noticed chest tightness one day at work, and whilst attending a stressful emergency experienced increasing pain. It developed to the point where his partner had to drive him to the local hospital, and it was discovered that he was suffering an acute heart attack. A stent (a small metal scaffold) was placed inside the blockage, thereby relieving it.

The man made an appointment to see me after this event, because he was perplexed. He ate the right foods, was extremely fit, had never smoked and had normal cholesterol and blood pressure levels.

Tests revealed that there was only one severe blockage, whilst the remainder of his arteries were very smooth, not suggesting blockages or any other irregularity. Because of the absence of risk factors, the man's young age and the fact that he had only one blockage with otherwise normal coronary arteries, I performed a test to determine whether he had a disorder which would predispose him to clotting. I found that he did.

In this case, the patient required emphasis on the management of his clotting tendency with blood-thinning agents like aspirin, rather than aggressive management of the more typical coronary risk factors such as high cholesterol. He remains well five years on.

CASE STUDY 2: ASPIRIN AND THIN BLOOD

A female in her late seventies was quite short of breath. She had no bleeding, bowel symptoms, abdominal pain, or change in appetite – only the shortness of breath and a moderate degree of fatigue.

I organised blood tests, which revealed that she was severely anaemic. I asked her about her medications and she gave me a list made up of the standard pot-pourri of pills ingested by many older members of the community. One of these included aspirin, which she took because she thought it was good for the heart.

A gastroscopy (when a tube is inserted through the mouth into the stomach) revealed that she had quite severe gastritis (inflammation of the stomach), a condition that is often associated with aspirin ingestion – because her blood was made thin by the aspirin, she bled from her inflamed stomach, causing her to lose half her blood volume.

'One size does not fit all' in aspirin use, as with all medications and medical procedures. I believe that people with thick blood should take aspirin daily, whilst people with thin blood should avoid it. The decision to take aspirin should be made after a thorough assessment of risk by your doctor.

CARDIOVASCULAR DISEASE

Cardiovascular disease (including heart disease and stroke) accounts for around 45 per cent of deaths in modern society, and this figure is not dropping significantly.

CAUSES OF CARDIOVASCULAR DISEASE

The traditionally quoted risk factors for heart disease include high cholesterol, high blood pressure, cigarette smoking, diabetes and having a strong family history of the disease. Over the past ten years, however, we have recognised that there are other major contributors; for example, psychosocial factors such as job strain, social isolation and depression are clearly associated with the risk of heart attack.

A recent study from *The New England Journal of Medicine* suggested that travelling in peak-hour traffic can increase your risk of a heart attack within one hour of exposure by anywhere between 250 and 400 per cent. The researchers involved in the study suggested that the problem might be caused by the combination of waking up in the morning, stress of being in the traffic itself, noise, and traffic-related air pollution.

The basic key to cardiovascular disease is modern living. Many aspects of our society are completely unnatural, but are accepted as part of life and play a strong part in our modern diseases.

Synthetic chemicals and stress both involve excessive use of oxygen. When the body is introduced to a synthetic chemical, more oxygen and energy are required to cope with it, as the body is designed to cope with only natural chemicals. When the body is stressed, the stress hormones that are released make the body work harder and more oxygen is consumed.

Oxygen is, of course, essential for our existence, but if we use too much, we generate free radicals, which erode the lining of the blood vessels and damage DNA, putting us at risk of heart disease and cancer. There are many other substances, such as lipoprotein (a) and homocysteine, that also aid the generation of excessive free radicals.

Risk factors for cardiovascular disease

Over the years there have been numerous novel risk factors reported for cardiovascular disease:

Childhood abuse

A recent US Government–funded study of around 17,000 people showed that those with a history of emotional abuse as a child had a 70 per cent higher chance of developing heart disease by the age of 50 than those who had a happy childhood. Being the victim of physical violence as a child increased the risk by around 50 per cent.

Growing up in a family with a history of mental illness, substance abuse or criminality was also cited as a risk factor.

Acute stress

For many years there has been conjecture as to the place of stress in the risk factors for cardiovascular disease.

I have long been a proponent of the association between stress and cardiovascular disease, but many conservative researchers state that stress has no bearing on its acceleration, progression or causation.

A study at St Vincent's Hospital in Melbourne looked at emotional stress as a heart attack risk. It considered case reports of three women aged from 40 to 58 who had suffered acute stress and had suffered heart attacks. It was felt that this particular stress induced coronary artery spasms, which led to the heart attacks. Fortunately, in each case the abnormalities in the heart resolved and subsequent angiograms were normal.

Weather

A recent study from France has shown that a sudden change in the weather leading to a cold snap may trigger an acute heart attack, especially if a person has underlying high blood pressure. The study followed 700 people over two years, and found that the occurrence of heart attacks in people with high blood pressure doubled when the average temperature was lower than –4 degrees Celsius.

It has been known for many years that changes in temperature, especially towards cold, cause acute spasm in the arteries, which can rupture plaques.

THE HEART AND ALTITUDE

It has long been known that people who live at high altitudes appear to have greater stamina than those who live at sea level. A recent study in Greece looked at three particular villages: two situated on the plains and one which was 1000 metres higher. The results showed that the people living at the high altitude had lower death rates from cardiovascular disease. It was felt that the lower oxygen concentration at this height forced the heart to work more efficiently.

However, a study from China showed that children born at a high altitude had far more occurrence of hole in the heart. A hole present at birth usually closes in time, but if it is not fed a large enough dose of oxygen it may remain open. We can't win, can we?

Prevention of cardiovascular disease

With an accurate, early preventative assessment (in the form of a simple questionnaire that involves obtaining a history of cholesterol abnormalities, high blood pressure, cigarette smoking, diabetes and a family history of the disease, especially before the age of 55) followed by lifestyle modification, appropriate antioxidant therapy and targeted treatment when necessary, it is my firm belief that around 90 to 95 per cent of cardiovascular disease can be prevented.

If we were prepared to put a greater effort into these preventative strategies, we could probably knock coronary artery bypass grafting off its position as the number one operation in our society (thousands of procedures are performed throughout the modern world on a weekly basis).

Surely the best treatment is prevention.

Treatment of cardiovascular disease

Coronary artery bypass grafting is an extremely effective lifesaving procedure in many cases of heart disease. Of course there is a small risk of death with any surgical procedure, and the more intensive that procedure, the greater the risk. Coronary artery bypass grafting is commonly complicated by other medical conditions. As with all aspects of medicine, the risks of the procedure must be weighed against its benefits.

The greatest risk factor for heart disease is having had heart disease in the first place. If you do not find the cause for your particular heart disease and treat that cause, the disease will recur in the grafted arteries on average within the next six to eight years.

In my opinion, anyone who has had coronary artery bypass grafting should visit a preventative cardiologist on a yearly basis, to ensure that the underlying atherosclerotic process is being treated aggressively.

CASE STUDY: CORONARY ARTERY BYPASS GRAFTING AND COMPLICATIONS

Former US president Bill Clinton recently underwent coronary artery bypass grafting, at the age of 58. An interesting question arose from his experience: why did such a young man have such a serious, life-threatening disease? The most obvious answer is the way in which Clinton has lived his life. He was the US president for eight years: an extremely stressful occupation. He was also a junk food aficionado for a long time and has cycled through weight gain and weight loss over a number of decades.

Just before his heart problems occurred, Clinton had lost a significant amount of weight on the South Beach diet. This is a sensible, high-protein, low-carbohydrate diet, but many of the diet's critics say that it contributed to Clinton's severe coronary disease. The reason given by the critics (and I disagree with this argument) is that the fat content of the South Beach Diet increases cholesterol and triglyceride levels in the blood stream, increasing the risk for heart disease. Dr Arthur Agatson, the author of The South Beach Diet book, is a well-respected cardiologist in America and has thoroughly researched the safety and efficacy of his diet. There is no foundation for the proposal that this diet adversely affects cholesterol levels or increases the risk for heart disease.

Clinton recovered extremely well from the bypass surgery but afterwards had a moderate complication that had nothing to do with his heart. Almost everybody who undergoes coronary artery bypass grafting has a degree of lung collapse after the operation and can develop fluid and scarring around the lung as a consequence of this collapse. This happened to Clinton, and he underwent a further operation to remove the fluid and scar tissue from his left lung.

Cholesterol and cardiovascular disease

Recently I saw a woman in her eighties who came into my consulting room nervously clutching her cholesterol results, seemingly fearful that I would either tell her she was in big medical trouble or suggest a pill to lower her cholesterol. This illustrates some important points regarding cholesterol:

- Over the past 20 to 30 years the public has been made unnecessarily concerned about the presence of cholesterol, which is an essential body chemical.
- Focusing on the total cholesterol result in blood tests is far too simplistic and in many cases misleading.
- The most important aspect of any case is you, not the blood test results.

On the surface, the case for cholesterol as a major risk for heart disease appears quite solid. In the late 1950s, Professor Ancel Keys introduced the notion of links between cholesterol, fat and heart disease in his Seven Countries Study, and since then the medical profession and pharmaceutical industry have 'run with the ball'. Most doctors and the general public have an unquestioning belief in the link between diet, cholesterol and the risk of heart attack. Over the past five years, however, a vocal minority has emerged questioning the importance of cholesterol and even the entire diet–heart hypothesis.

Although I believe the link is clear between diet and heart disease, I am not convinced that these are linked so strongly with total cholesterol. I believe the dietary culprits are trans (synthetic) fats and processed carbohydrates. Interestingly, over the past few years, some studies have suggested that the cholesterol link is only relevant in cases of heart disease up to the age of 50, and thereafter blood pressure elevation and smoking are much more important. I often see patients in my clinic over the age of 50 who are dutifully swallowing their statin drugs to lower their cholesterol levels, but have abysmal control of their blood pressure. I really can't see the sense in this approach.

I am in no way suggesting that cholesterol should be ignored, but it appears to be a greater concern for doctors and patients than blood pressure and, in my view, this is the wrong way around.

EXERCISE AND CARDIOVASCULAR DISEASE

An interesting study from the *Journal of the American Medical Association* showed that it is more important to be fit than it is to be thin. This study said that the risk of heart disease is significantly higher in those who are unfit when compared with those who are overweight. So, regardless of what the scales say, we need to get out there and pound the pavement – and reap the long-term benefits.

CANCER

For as long as I can remember, the highest number of deaths in Western society has been from cardiovascular disease. The cardiac mortality on a yearly basis is roughly 45 per cent of all deaths, with cancer at around 30 per cent. Recently, however, projections have been released by the New South Wales Health Department suggesting that common cancers (including melanoma, colon, breast and prostate cancers) could rise by approximately 25 per cent by 2011.

Causes of common cancers

The reason for the increase in melanoma is excessive sun exposure. The increase in bowel, breast and prostate cancer is multifactorial, but I believe it is partly diet-related, with the rising dependency on processed, packaged food and subsequent obesity rates. I also believe there is a contribution made by exposure to synthetic chemicals. For more information on the causes of cancer, please refer to *The Cell Factor*.

Prevention of cancer

As with all diseases, the best treatment for any type of cancer is to prevent it in the first place, which involves persistent focus on a healthy lifestyle and specific interventions for particular cancers.

Melanoma

It is important to avoid sun exposure and have regular skin checks with an expert.

Colon

I am a strong advocate of all adults over the age of 40 having a colonoscopy at some stage. Polyps, which are small raised lesions in the wall of the bowel, are very common pre-cancerous tumours. The value of the colonoscopy is that these can be snared and removed during the diagnostic procedure. This has been shown to markedly reduce the risk of cancer at a later stage. I would also advocate regular checkups using a faecal occult blood test, which involves checking stools for blood.

A recent study from the *Journal of the National Cancer Institute* showed an interesting benefit of calcium supplementation: taking 1200 milligrams of calcium carbonate per day can reduce the risk of more advanced polyps going on to form cancers by around 35 per cent. As there are many other benefits from the ingestion of calcium, I believe this should therefore be taken as part of a sensible supplement regimen.

Breast

Regular breast screening, including self-examination, is suggested for all adult women. Most experts support the use of mammography in women aged from 50 to 70 years.

Controversies still remain over hormone replacement therapy, breastfeeding and the timing of pregnancy and the relationship to breast cancer.

Recent work from the *Journal of the American Medical Association* followed around 3000 women and showed that those who exercised for more than three hours per week had fewer occurrences of breast cancer by between 20 and 50 per cent compared with women who did less exercise.

Prostate

Again, there is controversy as to the place of PSA testing (Prostate Specific Antigen, a simple blood test) as a means of detecting early prostate cancer. The two best preventative strategies for prostate cancer are (1) use it or lose it – a simple principle for any health strategy is to use your organs for the function they are designed; and (2) regular digestion of lycopene-based foods such as cooked tomatoes.

Our basic survival mechanisms are being tested to the limit by modern diseases. We are seeing an epidemic of obesity and diabetes and, for the first time, cancer is seriously competing with cardiovascular disease as the most common cause of death. Although modern medicine and scientific research are moving closer to cures for these diseases (and there are already many effective treatments available), surely the best treatment for all of them is not to develop them in the first place.

Too often doctors see patients who don't want to take their medications or have surgical intervention, but unfortunately have allowed themselves to progress to the point where these measures are necessary. Years of exposure to processed, packaged foods, synthetic chemicals and chronic stress, along with reduced activity, have left their legacy in our bodies. Drugs are not all bad – some synthetically caused diseases will need a synthetic treatment. In many instances drugs have saved and prolonged lives. My real concern is the fact that people frequently wait until their diseases are firmly established before seeking appropriate medical supervision and therapy.

Lifestyle must be seen as the foundation of a long and healthy life. Pills, interventions or procedures must always be seen as a last resort rather than an easy solution. If we do not want convenience to be our killer, we must start thinking about how we can go back to a more natural style of living within the realm of our modern world. Part 2 will help us to begin the process.

CHAPTER 5

Modern medical and nutritional debates

In researching this book, I have come across many fascinating debates in medical and nutritional circles. This chapter contains outlines of those that the reader might find instructive, or simply interesting: cholesterol; problems with medical trials; milk and health; nutritional supplements; and tap water safety.

CHOLESTEROL

Think of the subtle psychology involved when someone is told they have 'high cholesterol'. The typical scenario lets both the doctor and the patient off the hook. The patient is told by the doctor that their cholesterol is elevated but that they mustn't panic, as there is a cure. There is a wonderful group of drugs known as statins. Simply by swallowing one of them once a day, their cholesterol levels can be superbly controlled. Thirty seconds later, the patient is out of the door with the prescription – and with no stern lectures about boring diets or arduous exercise programs. The patient thinks that they need not change their lifestyle, but simply swallow a pill every day.

It is my firm belief we should not treat or even consider for treatment an isolated cholesterol result. The more extensive lipid (total fat) profile should be the baseline test before treatment, but most government medical bodies and health insurance companies ignore this. However, your health is your responsibility so the next time a doctor suggests a cholesterol test, I would suggest asking for tests on:

- Cholesterol and triglycerides (HDL and BSL)
- Lipoprotein (a)
- Apolipoprotein B (Apo B) and Apolipoprotein A1 (Apo A1)
- High-sensitivity C-Reactive Protein (hsCRP)
- Homocysteine
- Fibrinogen

(The three tests at the end of the list are not part of the lipid profile, but are still important risk indicators for heart disease.) My reasons for suggesting these tests are as follows.

Cholesterol and triglycerides

Most people with an interest in health are aware that there are good and bad cholesterols. The bad is LDL; the good is HDL. Numerous studies have confirmed the importance of the cholesterol–HDL ratio as an accurate predictor of heart disease. This is why we should consider the entire fat (lipid) profile rather than looking at total cholesterol alone. LDL cholesterol puts fat into the artery walls, whereas HDL removes the fat from the walls. Thus, too much LDL is bad, but too little HDL is equally bad, hence the importance of the ratio.

Around 30 per cent of people with atherosclerotic heart disease have relatively normal total cholesterols but a low HDL, and therefore an abnormal ratio. Their risk of heart disease is just as high (possibly even more so) as an isolated, elevated cholesterol, and are much higher than for a person with an elevated cholesterol but also a high HDL (giving them a normal cholesterol–HDL ratio – the Acceptable Ratio is <3.5; the Ideal Ratio is <2.5). I am staggered by the number of people with high cholesterol and high HDL (therefore a normal ratio) who are prescribed statin drugs. Equally alarming are those whose total cholesterol might be approximately 5.2 but who have an HDL of 0.9, and who have been reassured by their doctor that their cholesterol is good and should be of no concern.

Much of this comes back to psychology: it is simple to treat high cholesterol but, at present, our available treatment for low HDL levels is not so straightforward. Apart from addressing a few lifestyle factors such as diet (increasing monounsaturated fats, reducing trans fats, consuming low-dose alcohol), regular exercise and smoking cessation, there are not many ways to raise HDL levels. Currently the only pharmaceutical preparation that lifts HDL is the old-style pharmaceutical-strength Niacin. In many countries there is a new preparation of Niacin, known as Niaspan-TM, which can be taken as a large, single dose at night and doesn't cause the marked flushing that is commonly seen with short-acting preparations. Nor does it have the liver toxicity of the older, slow-release preparations.

However, new drugs are now being trialled that specifically raise HDL levels. One of these is Torcetrabib. This drug has been shown in preliminary trials to raise HDL levels by around 50 per cent. It will be interesting to see how much impact the drug has on reducing heart attacks.

LDL, the bad cholesterol, is divided into two main types – small and dense, and large and buoyant. The large, buoyant type makes up the bulk of LDL cholesterol but is, in fact, nowhere near as important as the small, dense type, whose molecules are more easily attacked by free radicals and, once oxidised, are the major component of LDL cholesterol to pass across the blood vessel wall and set up fatty plaques.

In many countries, including Australia, LDL components cannot be measured. However, HDL and triglyceride levels give a good indication of whether a person has excess small LDL. If the triglycerides are elevated and/or the HDL is low, it is likely that small LDL is present in the blood stream, regardless of total cholesterol levels. Statin drugs don't have a major effect on this type of LDL cholesterol, and it is more effectively treated with a diet high in quality fats and proteins, and low in processed carbohydrates.

Lipoprotein (a)

As we saw in Chapter 3, this large, cholesterol-carrying molecule throws fat into the arteries and thickens the blood. If a person's lipoprotein (a) levels are elevated, their risk of heart disease is 70 per cent higher than those with normal levels.

Apolipoprotein

Apolipoprotein molecules are important: Apo B carries LDL cholesterol and Apo A1 carries HDL cholesterol. Apo B to Apo A1 ratios have recently been shown to be excellent predictors of cardiac risk.

High-sensitivity C-Reactive Protein

Over the past ten years or so, a blood test known as hsCRP (high-sensitivity C-Reactive Protein) has been well researched as a very sensitive indicator of inflammation. Inflammation has been shown to have an integral role in the generation of our major killers – heart disease (vascular disease), cancer and other chronic diseases such as Alzheimer's.

Professor Paul Ridker, a cardiologist from Harvard University, has led the world in the research of hsCRP. His work, confirmed by many other centres, has clearly shown that the higher the hsCRP, the higher your risk for all forms of chronic disease, especially vascular disease. The ranked levels of hsCRP are as follows.

hsCRP	Level of risk
0–1.5	Low
1.5–3	Mid range
3–4.5	High
>4.5	Very high

Homocysteine

It is my opinion that everyone should have their homocysteine levels assessed as part of any preventative assessment. Why? Because homocysteine levels are indicators of the efficacy of your methylation system – your cellular repair kit. The lower your homocysteine level, the more efficient the repair kit.

Homocysteine is created in the body from the essential amino acid (one of the chemicals that form proteins) known as methionine. Although there is a significant contribution to your H-level through genetics, lifestyle factors are also very important. And here is where the age-old concept of balance is so vital: a diet high in protein (e.g. animal fats) without taking in high-quality B Group vitamins to break down homocysteine in the body, will tip the balance towards excessive homocysteine production. This toxic amino acid is delighted to tear your arterial lining (known as the endothelium) to shreds, allowing any excessive fat to spill into your artery walls (called atherosclerosis). Just for good measure, homocysteine also damages platelets, making them sticky and thus forming clots within the arterial channel. These are two things you certainly don't want to happen!

However, if you have a balanced diet in which you consume adequate protein but also ingest foods or supplements high in B Group vitamins (such as folate), the theory is that homocysteine levels can be lowered, along with your risk of cardiovascular disease. (Although there is yet to be a published trial that clearly and definitively demonstrates that lowering homocysteine with multivitamins reduces your risk of vascular disease, it is accepted that if your homocysteine is elevated, you are at higher risk for all manner of vascular events.)

Fibrinogen

Fibrinogen is a non-specific indicator of blood thickness. Levels of fibrinogen above 4 indicate a higher risk for cardiovascular events.

The *you* factor is the most important of all when considering what to do about abnormal lipid profiles. Your medical history and life situation is the most relevant in determining the management of your overall fat (lipid) profile.

A disturbing trend in modern times is the push to screen cholesterol levels in young people. Although I am a great advocate of all manner of testing and of prevention, I am an even greater advocate of common sense; we have recently witnessed the hazards of treating children with antidepressant agents. If screening must be done at an early age, I believe it is absurd to take a child or a teenager with mid-range cholesterol levels and even consider prescribing a statin drug to lower them. Instead, young people with raised cholesterol should follow a balanced lifestyle program such as the one set out later in this book.

MEDICAL TRIALS

This section aims to demonstrate the flaws in the scientific method of medical trials, using hormone replacement therapy (HRT), whose rise and fall over the past ten to 15 years has been one of the interesting trends in modern medicine, as an example.

When medical science investigates any pill, potion or procedure for risk or benefit, there is a standard approach. Firstly and most importantly comes the hypothesis, which is based on some scientific presumptions. The hypothesis for HRT suggested that the symptoms of menopause, such as hot flushes, mood swings, depression and the most obvious – cessation of periods – were related to ovarian failure.

The function of the ovaries is to produce eggs, as well as the oestrogen and progesterone that enable and maintain pregnancy. In addition, the ovaries regulate the monthly female cycle to prepare a woman during her reproductive years for a possible pregnancy. A number of beneficial effects are attributed to oestrogen, and these form the basis of the HRT benefit hypothesis:

- Oestrogen is one of the body's natural vasodilators, which means it opens up blood vessels and helps to keep the blood pressure low.
- In natural doses, oestrogen released from the ovaries has a beneficial effect on blood clotting and cholesterol.
- Oestrogen maintains healthy bones and the elasticity of the skin.

The oestrogen hypothesis – so popular back in the late 1980s and early 1990s – suggested that supplying oestrogen to peri-menopausal women would not only create a reduction in symptoms, but would also reduce occurrence of common diseases such as heart disease, cancer and osteoporosis.

Once the hypothesis has a plausible scientific basis, and this one certainly did, it is tested at a number of levels. The first and second levels of scientific proof are laboratory and animal evidence. Oestrogen passed these tests. The third level is the observation and epidemiology trials. In these, populations or communities of peoples are tested, examined and followed, usually for a number of years, to determine their characteristics and response to different interventions.

The 'holy grail' of medicine is the randomised, controlled, double-blinded clinical trial. This medical mouthful means that a number of people at risk of a condition are selected, and the people who don't want to be in the study (usually a large number) and those who will adversely affect the results (because they have some other, unrelated condition that could prematurely interrupt their existence) are excluded.

The remaining subjects are followed for a period (usually around five years), with half receiving the active treatment being trialled and the other half a sugar pill (placebo). At the end of the study period the results will be processed, and are usually presented in the best possible light for the pill, potion or procedure (often because the company producing the medication paid for the trials).

The Nurses Health Study in Boston, which has been in action for the past 25 years, is one of the trials that has suggested strong benefits from HRT. This trial reported around a 50 per cent reduction in cardiovascular disease in those nurses taking HRT, with similar reductions in osteoporosis. There was a small but insignificant rise in breast cancer in the nurses taking HRT. The Nurses Health Study did not use the randomised method, but carried out the tests as an observational trial, a type of test that does not select any pill, potion or procedure but purely watches, and then analyses the resulting data. The researchers assessed how many of the nurses in the study were taking HRT regularly, either through their own choice or on the advice of their doctor, and compared them with nurses in a comparable peri-menopausal age range who weren't taking HRT. They were followed for a number of years to determine heart disease, osteoporosis and breast cancer rates.

Because self-selection can change results, observational trials are never accepted as final evidence by the medical scientific community. The argument for this approach is that a woman who seeks HRT and is prepared to swallow the treatment long-term may be more 'health motivated' in other ways, and this could affect the results. HRT users were, in fact, found to eat more healthily, exercise more, take more vitamins and smoke less than non-users.

Two recent trials reviewed in prestigious medical journals that did use the randomised method have turned the entire HRT debate on its head. Both suggested a marked increase in heart attack, stroke and thromboses, with a small but definite increase in breast cancer rates in post-menopausal women who had been given oestrogen. As soon as these trials were released, droves of HRT users stopped taking their treatment. Many women felt cheated by the entire medical process, and this has contributed to the increasing mistrust of many of the medical messages transmitted with confidence by the profession to the public.

The two randomised trials of HRT were not carried out on peri-menopausal women – the group that actually may benefit from this therapy. Instead, the trials focused on women who were, on average, post-menopausal by 15 to 18 years. A female body goes through definite stages, and something that works at one stage may have the opposite effect at another. Whether HRT is safe for peri-menopausal women and whether it prevents or contributes to common diseases in these women has not been proved or disproved. All that is known at present is that it should not be started in a woman who is over 15 years post-menopause.

So, are randomised trials trustworthy? Should we only listen to the results of these trials and ignore all other medical evidence? Although it is laudable to demand absolute scientific proof for all aspects of life, it will never be available, because we are all different, and cannot expect similar lives or similar reactions to diets, exercise, or drugs. So when large numbers of people are grouped together for the purpose of a medical study, the variations between them are such that we can only expect variable results. With ever increasing amounts of scientific knowledge available, it is not surprising that confusing results occur.

COW'S MILK: POISON OR POTION?

As with all aspects of nutrition, medicine and pharmacology, there are varying opinions, vested interests, and needs for disclosures on this subject. For many years, conservative nutritionists and preventative cardiologists have pushed the low-fat, 'keep the dairy to a bare minimum' line. Over the past five to ten years, however, evidence has increasingly emerged to suggest that this message may be too simplistic.

MILK AND DISEASE

Recent work supervised by Professor Julie Campbell from the University of Queensland has demonstrated that a major determinant of milk-related cardiovascular disease is the type of protein in the milk rather than the fat content. Milk proteins are divided into those that are soluble, known as the whey proteins, and those that are insoluble (or more solid), the caseins. Caseins make up just over 80 per cent of the total proteins, whereas whey proteins form about 5 per cent.

The study showed that there are two distinct insoluble milk proteins – beta-casein A1 and beta-casein A2 – the first being pro-atherogenic (promotes the build-up of fat in the walls of arteries) and the other, anti-atherogenic (prevents the build-up). From this it is logical to assume, although not yet proved, that milk containing more beta-casein A2, the anti-atherogenic protein, may help to prevent the risk of heart disease.

Milk that has a higher proportion of A1 than A2 has been linked to the following conditions:

Atherosclerotic heart disease

A 20-year study involving 20 countries demonstrated a clear link between the consumption of high-A1 milk and this common type of heart disease. Finland, Ireland and New Zealand had the highest rates of heart disease deaths (between 300 and 400 deaths per 100,000 people), and France and Japan had the lowest rates (between 50 and 100 deaths per 100,000). People in the first group of countries consumed around three to five grams of high-A1 milk per day, equivalent to consuming 250 millilitres of pure A1. People in the second group consumed less than one gram of high-A1 milk per day.

Interestingly, when examining cardiac risk factors in Belfast, Ireland, and Toulouse, France, there were almost identical results in cholesterol levels, blood pressure and smoking rates. The only real differences between the two cities were the intake of high-A1 milk and the rate of heart disease, both of which were three times higher in Belfast.

Diabetes

Studies have shown a strong link between A1 proteins and the risk of insulin-dependent (also called Type I or juvenile onset) diabetes.

Autism

A small but vocal group of researchers and clinicians are firmly convinced of a link between A1 protein and autism. A study of 81 children with autism demonstrated that 95 per cent of them had a level of milk protein in their blood and urine that was 100 times higher than the normal level. Professor Robert J Cade of the University of Florida stated that when these children were put on a milk-free diet, 80 per cent had a reduction of their symptoms. Many of the characteristics of autism were markedly reduced, improving over six to 12 months. As the levels of milk protein were so high in the blood and urine of most of the children with autism, they might indeed have suffered from mechanisms that were defective in handling the A1 protein.

Please note that milk with high A2 content is just as allergenic as milk with high A1, and both types of milk should be avoided by people with a milk allergy. In Australia, the typical milk purchased (regardless of the fat content) is a mix of around 60 per cent A2 and 40 per cent A1. Therefore, on balance, Australian milk is beneficial and regular consumption should be encouraged.

Some cows are now being bred to produce close to 100 per cent A2 milk, which is now available in Australia. Interestingly, the Masai people of Kenya consume large quantities of milk from Zebu cows, which produce 98 per cent A2 milk. The Masai have very low rates of atherosclerosis.

Milk and bone health

Recently a meta-analysis of 47 studies showed little relationship between calcium intake and bone health in children. The study suggested that the major factor in maintaining strong bones was regular exercise.

I am always disappointed when I read studies like these, as I believe they focus too much on one or two aspects of a disease process. For this meta-analysis the studies that were featured focused specifically on calcium intake in childhood and bone health. They were mostly short-term, and did not look at anything higher than the 15- to 20-year effects of high versus low calcium intake from dairy products.

In my opinion, when the weight of evidence is examined, dairy products should be encouraged in children and adults, and not just from the perspective of bone health. There is also now very elegant work to demonstrate that people who are encouraged to consume dairy products as children have lower rates of late-onset diabetes.

The most concerning aspect for me is that if we demean the benefits of dairy products, children will continue to consume cola-based drinks, which have been shown to actively remove calcium from the bones and increase the risk of bone fractures in teenagers. We are now also seeing younger people with significant osteoporosis.

On balance, for all the reasons stated, the regular consumption of milk should be encouraged, not avoided. Furthermore, I am unconvinced that low-fat varieties of milk offer much of a health benefit (if at all) over the standard, full-cream products.

ANTIOXIDANT SUPPLEMENTS

If you believe conservative health care professionals, you will think that all vitamin supplements do is give you expensive urine. However, I am a strong believer in the regular ingestion of appropriate doses of combined, natural supplementation.

The best known antioxidants are vitamins C and E. It is my opinion that a person who is over 35 years old should take, on a daily basis, 1000 milligrams of vitamin C and 250 to 500 international units (IU) of vitamin E (d-alpha tocopherol – the natural version), preferably at night. (The synthetic version of vitamin E, dl-alpha tocopherol, should not be used.) Night is the recommended time to take these supplements because it is when we usually take in our greatest food load. Also, our livers tend to produce more fat in the evening.

NEW ANTIOXIDANT SUPPLEMENTS

There is now a group of new-generation antioxidants reported to be much more powerful than vitamins C and E. The group includes substances such as Coenzyme Q10, alpha lipoic acid, and grape seed and pine bark extracts. Whether there is an added benefit from taking these instead of or as well as vitamins E and C is a matter of conjecture. If you believe the conservatives, you are wasting your money with all of them. If you are more convinced by testimonials, the manufacturers of any of these substances will be able to produce people willing to say how the supplements have given them anything from greater energy to a cure for cancer.

As with most aspects of life, I believe the answer lies somewhere in the middle. There is no miracle drug, procedure or supplement.

Vitamin E

Many practitioners in the complementary world are convinced of the health benefits of vitamin E, but a recent meta-analysis from the *Annals of Internal Medicine* actually suggested that taking vitamin E in high doses could increase the risk of death. The paper which presented this theory is entitled *Vitamin E meta-analysis – Vitamin E may increase all-cause mortality*. I believe it speaks volumes about the way that medical research is coducted around the world and, in particular, how conservative medicine approaches the research of complementary therapies.

The researchers at Johns Hopkins University analysed 19 previously performed studies of vitamin E therapy. Eleven of these were studies where daily vitamin E doses that were greater than 400 IU were used. The results of these studies showed that there were 39 more deaths per 10,000 people than in those who took a placebo. This just reached statistical significance. Interestingly, in those who ingested a low dose of vitamin E (less than 400 IU per day) there were 16 fewer deaths.

Regardless of the conclusions of the study, I believe the analysis was flawed and should be completely disregarded, a view that I will justify below.

Not all vitamin E is created equal. The commonly used versions of the vitamin for supplementation are dl-alpha tocopherol (the synthetic version) and d-alpha tocopherol (the natural version). The latter is more expensive, so isn't normally used in clinical trials.

Many of the studies involved in the meta-analysis were analysing supplementary use of vitamin E alone, not a combination of vitamins. The use of sole vitamins in antioxidant doses (which are much higher than the recommended daily allowance) has no scientific validity or common sense, as antioxidants, both in the body and in food, are always found in combination with a mix of antioxidant chemicals. In fact, if we use a sole antioxidant such as vitamin E (especially the cheaper, lower standard versions of it), we can potentially do more harm than good, because the vitamin E is quickly overwhelmed by free radicals and becomes a pro-oxidant (a free radical).

Therefore the only possible way that supplemental vitamins can be of benefit is if they are taken in combination with other high-quality antioxidant preparations. In this meta-analysis there were only three studies that used a combination of antioxidant vitamins, and in all of these, synthetic vitamins were used, rendering the studies useless.

Statistics can be presented in any way to suit your argument. In the United States (unlike Australia), there is no government sponsorship of pharmaceutical agents, so individuals have to pay for their drugs as well as their vitamins. Therefore, there is direct competition between the pharmaceutical industry and the vitamin industry for the health dollar.

All of the studies performed on vitamins carry heavy

sponsorship from the pharmaceutical industry. It is in the interest of the pharmaceutical companies to prove that vitamin supplements don't work, and they have succeeded. The scientific world is now saying that there is no point in studying vitamins further because they obviously don't work and, in fact, are probably harmful. No single vitamin company will be able to sponsor a large trial of high-quality combination vitamins over the required ten-year period, yet this is what is needed to demonstrate a benefit in the general population.

When someone is a subject in a clinical trial, they are put into either the active treatment group or the placebo group. If, for some reason, a person stops taking the active treatment or moves from the placebo group to the active treatment group, on paper, they remain in their initial group.

In the Chaos trial performed in Cambridge, England, there was said to be a slight increase in deaths in those taking vitamin E compared with those taking a placebo, but the vitamin group experienced a 77 per cent reduction in non-fatal heart attacks. This information seems incredibly contradictory, but when we look closely, we find that during the two-year study there were only six deaths in people taking vitamin E, and 72 deaths in people not taking vitamin E. Unfortunately, many of the vitamin E group had stopped taking the supplement, and these were the ones who suffered a cardiac-related death. Because they were initially in the vitamin E group, they were still included in that group for the results, although they weren't taking vitamin E at the time of their death.

There was no real emphasis on lifestyle modification

during the trials. This meant that the vitamins were used as drugs, not supplements to a healthy lifestyle.

If you look at all the indirect evidence from laboratory work, animal experimentation and epidemiology, and weed out the important information from the best of the randomised clinical trials, I believe there is overwhelming proof that we should be taking high-quality pharmaceutical-grade vitamins in combination for a prolonged period.

Vitamin C

Over the past 20 years there have been numerous clinical trials of vitamin C therapy, some positive and some negative in their results. A recent review from the Nurses Health Study (mentioned above) showed a 27 per cent reduction in cardiac events in those nurses who regularly took high doses of supplemental vitamin C. A few years ago, however, a study from San Diego suggested that regular ingestion of the vitamin actually thickened arteries, a marker for future vascular events, and so recommended that vitamin C ingestion should be avoided.

The problems with the San Diego trial are the same as those for vitamin E. They didn't include lifestyle modification, and there were such varying doses and preparations used that much of the information is difficult to interpret. I believe that there is benefit from taking combination vitamins and, as stated above, vitamin E and vitamin C taken together at night are of significant benefit for reducing the risk of vascular disease.

Benefits of vitamin C supplementation

- Vitamin C is a very important aspect of collagen formation.
- Under times of stress our vitamin C requirements increase.
- Vitamin C is involved in many aspects of our immune system.
- Vitamin C plays an important part in the overall antioxidant package in the body.
- Vitamin C is vital for the normal production of neurotransmitters, which are the chemical messengers involved in brain function.
- Vitamin C is also vital in the production of hormones, in iron absorption and in many other cellular processes.

Who should take vitamin C?

If you are under 35 years old, without any major illnesses, and not in a high-risk category for serious diseases later in your life, I can see no real benefit in supplementation. If you are over the age of 35 but have limited risk factors for heart disease or cancer, you are still at low risk and may only gain a minor benefit from vitamin C supplementation. If you are in a high-risk category for any major disease or already have an established major disease then I believe that vitamin C supplementation is of benefit.

Recommended doses of vitamin C

- Healthy, low-risk population over 35 years: 500–1000 milligrams per day

- Heart disease and cancer sufferers: 1–2 grams per day
- Special circumstances (for example, raised lipoprotein (a) levels): 2 grams per day

Anyone wishing to take high doses (greater than 1000 mg) should only do so under the recommendation and supervision of an expert health care professional.

TAP WATER SAFETY

We are encouraged to drink plenty of water and, if you believe the authorities (and they may be correct), our modern water supply is quite safe. But even the authorities wouldn't dispute that there are small amounts of chemicals, such as chlorine, fluoride and xenon, in drinking water. Because of the possible problems created by these chemicals, and concerns about bacteria, many people in modern Western cities use some form of filtration system. There are widely differing views on the necessity for this, ranging from the belief that our water supply is absolutely safe, with bottled water and filtration systems being one of many cons used to trick gullible, concerned citizens, to the belief that tap water is partly responsible not only for chronic gastrointestinal disturbances but also for contributing to heart disease and cancer.

So, what is the correct answer? I don't know. The problem with implicating that the water supply has an unbeneficial effect on our health is the vastness and availability of water along with the enormous amount of variables associated with modern disease. One of the major themes of this book is our exposure to many and varied synthetic chemicals. Our water supply is one potential source (amongst many) of small doses of synthetic chemicals. To implicate this one source is scientifically very difficult.

Certainly, you can prove in laboratory experiments that chlorine promotes atherosclerosis (fat build-up in the arteries) and diminishes vitamin E effect. And in the test tube, fluoride does affect bone metabolism and promote tumour growth in laboratory animals, but this does not necessarily mean we can jump to the conclusion that, when consumed in low doses from the water supply, these substances will do the same things in humans.

I do know that dehydration is bad for the body. I believe we should drink a reasonable amount of water (1–1.5 litres) throughout the day and that we should not overdo drinks that have a diuretic effect, such as those containing alcohol or caffeine, or that have excessive amounts of sugar, such as soft drinks and commercial fruit juices.

If you are worried about the quality of your tap water, drink bottled or filtered water. It's your decision!

PART 2

REDRESSING THE BALANCE THROUGH BODY TYPING

CHAPTER 6

Health essentials

One of the areas where 'convenience is killing us' is in the field of nutrition. There are two main aspects to sensible nutrition:

FOOD QUALITY

The bizarre nature of Western humanity means that no-one would purchase a car and put sand, gravel or mud in the tank and expect it to work, but many people are happy to swallow all kinds of synthetic, processed, packaged food and drink rather than high-quality fresh varieties, expecting their bodies to function well on this low-quality 'fuel'. We seem content to neglect (or even damage) our most valuable asset, our bodies, but only use the best quality, expensive petrol for our cars.

The quality of the food we eat is a vital consideration if we want good health. Natural, fresh food is the best kind that we can give our bodies.

CALORIE INTAKE

Almost everyone in modern Western society eats too much. Food is a central aspect of our lives, and much of our advertising is geared towards enticing us to eat. The multinational food companies able to afford prime-time television advertisements are usually pushing high-calorie, low-nutrition products rather than healthy, natural kinds.

We find it inconvenient to be hungry, to be dissatisfied with a meal or not completely filled up by it, resulting in the explosion of 'super-size' meals, which contain far more calories than we actually need.

We are eating larger amounts more frequently than our hunter-gatherer ancestors. Their total calorie intake was probably somewhere between 1000 and 1500 calories per day, whereas the average person living in modern Western society consumes around 2000 to 3000 calories daily.

The journal *Scientific American* reported that in tests carried out on mice, it was found that their life span lengthened from 39 to 56 months when their calorie intake was reduced. For humans, whilst under-nourishment is definitely not beneficial, reducing our calorie consumption can help us to live longer, avoiding heart disease, diabetes and cancer. This is because cutting back on the calories reduces free radical production which, as we have seen, is the central cause of all our modern diseases.

HEALTH PRINCIPLES

Simply reducing the amount of food we eat is not the way to achieve optimum health, however. Below are five basic principles for healthy eating and weight loss.

THE IN/OUT PRINCIPLE

The most important principle of weight loss is to consume less energy (in terms of daily intake) than you burn off.

Our bodies were designed to be hunter-gatherers who had to move around to find food and survive on much less of it than we do now. With our modern conveniences of readily available food sources and mechanical forms of transport, we are consuming more energy than we are burning. So instead of expending, we are expanding!

THE CONVENIENCE PRINCIPLE

The more food is processed, the fewer nutritional benefits it contains. Foods to avoid include:

Long-life food

If the food can be kept in a box, piece of plastic or container, in a thickened, hardened state with a use-by date, it is not good for you. Think about it. This degree of preservation comes at a serious cost. To keep the food in this state, in almost all cases there has to be small but definite quantities of trans fatty acids and other unnatural chemicals.

So, what do these trans fats do? They do to the cells of your body exactly what they do to the food: they thicken and harden the cells to reduce the normal entry of nutrients into the cell. The nutrients, in the form of fat, sugar and protein, no longer find it easy to get into the cells that need them, such as the vital organs and the muscles, but are soaked up by fat cells and get stuck in the lining of blood vessels to create that well-known process called atherosclerosis, still just edging out cancer as our number one killer.

So, a basic principle is that if it's in a box, a container or a sealed plastic bag, try to avoid it as much as possible (and this includes breakfast cereal). Or, better yet, go down to your local hire place, get yourself a blow torch and set the pantry on fire. (Of course, I'm not being serious. What is serious is the fact that regularly consuming long-life food is a slow form of suicide.)

Bakery food

Anything from bagels, croissants and doughnuts to bread rolls and white bread bombards our bodies with large doses of trans fats and processed carbohydrates, and contains little in the way of micro-nutrients.

Take-away food

These days, many families have more take-away meals than they have meals cooked at home. With the increasing need for double-income families, neither partner feels like cooking when they arrive home from a busy day and the convenient option is to order a take-away. Almost all take-away food has trans fats, processed carbohydrates and a fair amount of salt.

Sweet food

How sweet it isn't: low-fat foods leave a large hole in our taste experience, which has been replaced with sugar. If something says 'low fat' on the packet you can guarantee it's either full of sugar or salt. Something has to be in it to make you enjoy it. Remember, every piece of convenience comes at a price. All sweet foods are obviously sugar-based – that's why they're sweet! They are also one of the major reasons that we're seeing epidemics of diabetes and obesity.

White food

Total white-out: the simple principle here is that if the food is white (or close to it), it's probably not that good for you. This includes white rice, pasta, bread, and potato. I'm not saying that you need to avoid these foods completely, but consumption should be minimised.

The Paleolithic principle

Food that can be killed and eaten straightaway or grown in the garden (without processing) contains the most nutrients of any available food. There is really nothing simpler than this principle. Our bodies were designed for natural food.

THE 19 OUT OF 21 PRINCIPLE

Given the choice, I'm sure any hunter-gatherer would plunge themselves headlong into a Western lifestyle. One of the benefits they would enjoy would be the wide variety of tasty foods available. So this principle allows us to have two meals a week in which we eat whatever we like. Prohibition rarely works, and is a major reason why diets fail.

THE MOVEMENT PRINCIPLE

It is not possible to be healthy or maintain any sort of weight-loss program without regular movement and exercise. Not only will exercise reduce the risk of cardiovascular disease by around 30 per cent, but there is also recent work that shows a similar reduction in many types of cancer. I do not believe there is an option for diet *or* exercise; instead, it is important to have both a healthy eating program *and* a healthy exercise and movement program.

BASIC DIETARY REQUIREMENTS

This list contains the nutrients that humans need for optimum health. It is vital to include all of them in our diet.

FIBRE

The recommended daily intake (RDI) is 25–30 g per day. We obtain dietary fibre from fruits, vegetables, whole grains and legumes.

Fats

The RDI of fats (up to 30–40 per cent of daily caloric intake) is 40–80 g for males; 30–60 g for females, and 80–120 g for athletes/people who are very physically active.

Recommended foods containing fats include olive oil, avocados, nuts, fish, meat, poultry and dairy products. You should avoid processed, packaged foods, bakery items and take-away food.

High-quality proteins

An adequate but not excessive intake of high-quality proteins is vital for normal existence. The RDI is 0.8 g per kg of healthy body weight (20 per cent of total caloric intake). Severe protein deficiencies are only seen in very malnourished people and certainly do not occur in anyone who eats a normal Western diet. I still believe, however, that we are eating less protein than we should.

Recommended proteins are fish, nuts, mushrooms, eggs and natural soy products.

Unprocessed, complex carbohydrates

Although there is, as yet, no specific RDI for carbohydrates, the average intake is usually around 200 g per day. The maximum intake of simple sugars should be only 50 g. (For example, one teaspoon of sugar is 5 g of carbohydrate, and one can of soft drink is 50 g of carbohydrate, i.e. your maximum RDI in one hit.)

Complex carbohydrates are the larger polysaccharides that are either digestible starches (amylose and amylopectin) and the indigestible polysaccharides (the aforementioned dietary fibre).

The more natural the carbohydrate, the better it is for you. Therefore try to consume carbohydrates that have not been processed. If you enjoy bread, for example, have a couple of slices of wholegrain or brown bread per day. No matter what type of carbohydrate is consumed, it will eventually end up as sugar in the body and so we should not over-consume any type. Try to use wholegrain pasta, and either Basmati or brown rice. The best source of complex carbohydrates are fruits and vegetables.

Micro-nutrients

It is important to consume vitamins, minerals and trace metals on a daily basis. The more fresh and unprocessed the food is, the more of these micro-nutrients will be contained within it. All of the natural foods, including plant-based foods and animal and marine products, are rich sources of micronutrients.

DESIGNING A PROGRAM FOR LIFE

In the following chapters, the Walker Lifestyle Program is explained. Rather than being just a diet, it encourages you to adapt your whole way of living to a more natural style. As I argue in Chapter 7, diets alone don't work. It is important to consider all of the following aspects of lifestyle when designing a program that brings about optimum weight and better health:

- Achieving ideal body weight
- Body and muscle tone
- Energy levels
- Lack of cravings and persistent hunger
- Overall sense of wellbeing

When adopting any type of lifestyle change, taking small steps one at a time can add up to the complete success of your program. However, the most important steps occur at the beginning, and are taken in the mind.

Decision

You must decide if losing weight and eating healthily is what you really want. You must be aware of what, when, how, where and why you are eating. You must change your attitude to food and then commit yourself to the long haul.

Awareness

Once you've made the decision, start to monitor your eating habits. Become an observer of your own behaviour. What unnecessary foods do you consume during the day? Are you eating purely for comfort or to ward off depression or loneliness? Examine the aspects of your life that are stopping you from achieving your goals.

Often it's the little things during the day that add up. You develop the habit of eating a biscuit, doughnut or low-fat muffin with morning coffee, or snacking on foods during the mid-afternoon fatigue period when you need a lift or having some comfort chocolate as a treat just before bedtime.

Attitudinal shift

Now that you've recognised the limiting behaviours, it is time to start creating a new pattern of thinking. Instead of the morning doughnut, plan ahead so you have on hand some nuts, a piece of fruit, or even a protein bar or shake. This will fill the 'hole' without doing any harm.

Long-term commitment

Once you have performed an act for 30 days, it becomes a habit. So you only need to be disciplined for around a month for your new attitudes and behaviours to become automatic.

There is nothing temporary about changing your life for the better. Without permanent, lifelong change, you will continue to make the same mistakes with diet and lifestyle. Decide what you really want, and what you need to do to achieve that goal. Then start to make some permanent changes.

CHAPTER 7

Diets don't work

A simple principle of life is that if there are many solutions for a problem, then none of them can work that well. This is demonstrated clearly in the field of diets: just look at how many dietary books there are. Basically, diets don't work.

Why do people go on diets? Most often because they are trying to lose weight. But how many people do you know who have successfully lost weight and kept it off on a long-term basis? I expect the answer is either very few or none.

A recent trial in the 5 January 2005 edition of *The Journal of the American Medical Association* examined the efficacy of the four most popular diets in modern society.

The diets studied were:

- Atkins diet – high-fat, low-carbohydrate
- Ornish diet – ultra low-fat (similar to Pritikin)
- Zone diet – low glycaemic load
- Weight Watchers diet – calorie-restricted

The researchers followed 160 overweight people for 12 months. Within the group studied, the average body mass index (weight in kilograms divided by height in metres squared; see figure below) was 35, there was equal sex distribution, and the average age was around 50 years. The weight loss for all four diets was modest – on average around three kilograms. There was no difference in outcome between the diets. In those who lost weight, there were reductions in cholesterol levels, blood pressure, and C-reactive protein. The greatest benefits were seen in the people who completed the programs. The Ornish diet was finished by 50 per cent of the subjects, Atkins by 52 per cent, and Zone and Weight Watchers by 65 per cent.

So can we say that any of the four diets actually work? We will look at each in turn.

BMI = WEIGHT (KILOGRAMS) ÷ HEIGHT (METRES)^2	
<20	Underweight
20–26	Normal
26–30	Overweight
>30	Obese
>40	Morbidly obese

THE ATKINS DIET

After years of being told that low-fat diets are the best and healthiest way to lose weight, we continue to believe this. Despite the proven ineffectiveness of the low-fat approach, conservative medical and nutritional bodies still push this line and the widespread availability of low-fat foods is a testament to this disordered thinking.

The most powerful fat-burning diet available is the one devised by Dr Robert Atkins in the 1970s. He was the pioneer of the high-protein, high-fat, low-carbohydrate diet, of which there have been many spin-offs since. These diets have divided the nutritional world, with some experts suggesting that the high-protein, high-fat approach is the only sensible nutritional intervention, whilst the more conservative experts say the diets are the work of the devil.

In the 1970s Atkins, a cardiologist then in his thirties, looked in the mirror and did not like what he saw. He was overweight, had multiple chins and felt he could not morally or ethically instruct his patients to follow a healthy lifestyle if he could not do so himself. He felt that the low-fat message promoted by many august bodies such as the American Heart Association was just not working. He had read a research paper on the fat-burning benefits of a high-protein, high-fat, low-carbohydrate diet. He wrote a book, *Dr Atkins' Diet Revolution*, which achieved reasonable popularity but, as with many dietary fads, it soon became overwhelmed by the standard low-fat message.

In the 1990s Atkins re-emerged, this time as a major celebrity in the dietary world, with his diet seen as a real alternative to the low-fat message. Many celebrities jumped on the Atkins bandwagon, demonstrating marked, rapid weight loss. The Atkins phenomenon exploded and Atkins himself became a multi-millionaire, promoting his books, nutritional supplements and foods such as protein and snack bars that are based around his dietary concepts.

My problem with Atkins' message is that it is far too extreme. During the first few months of the program, to kick-start the fat-burning process, the amount of carbohydrates consumed is markedly reduced, which leads to the induction of a state of ketosis (which is one of the body's processes for the metabolism of body fat). Although most people can tolerate ketosis without any short-term harm and the diet certainly does start off the weight-loss program, I still have concerns, which I will outline below.

Soon after commencing the Atkins program, many people notice significant gastrointestinal problems including constipation, abdominal pain and at times even haemorrhoids. The marked reduction in carbohydrate consumption also means that fewer fruits and vegetables (nature's best form of carbohydrate) are eaten. This leads to a significant decrease in the intake of natural fibre, vitamins and phyto-chemicals. Atkins countered this by suggesting supplementary fibre, vitamins, minerals and trace metals. Although I'm a great believer in supplements, they should never be seen as replacement for the real thing – that's why they are called supplements!

In older people or those at risk of cardiovascular disease, the rapid fat-burning state induced by the Atkins diet can actually contribute to a heart attack or stroke in some people. This does not often happen, but it is certainly a tragedy when a health intervention such as a particular diet contributes to a major cardiovascular event.

The Atkins diet can also be harmful for people with a significant underlying medical disorder such as kidney impairment.

CASE STUDY: ATKINS DIET AND DISEASE

A 55-year-old man with long-standing diabetes and heart disease also suffered from significant abdominal obesity and marked impairment in kidney function. He decided to try the Atkins diet after hearing glowing testimonials about its efficacy in weight loss.

Within a week, the man's kidney function had deteriorated dramatically, to the point that if he had continued on the diet, he would have needed dialysis within a few weeks. This is because patients with significant kidney impairment cannot tolerate the higher protein load of the Atkins diet, or any of the related high-protein diets.

I'm not suggesting the Atkins diet causes kidney disease, but if a person has an underlying disease (even if only relatively mild), the diet may worsen their condition. The major problem here is that a small proportion of people lead normal lives unaware that they have kidney problems. They may commence a program such as Atkins' and within a few weeks could be in serious trouble.

If a person is young, overweight but otherwise healthy, and has been cleared by a doctor, the Atkins diet or an Atkins-style program may be the most effective method of rapid weight loss for them, but it is important to be aware that the long-term effects in large populations are as yet untested.

An alternative, far more moderate high-protein, high-fat, low-carbohydrate diet is Arthur Agatston's South Beach diet, which has recently taken the United States by storm.

THE ORNISH DIET

At the other end of the diet spectrum are programs developed by people like Nathan Pritikin and Dean Ornish, who push the ultra low-fat diets. In a study released in the 1990s, Ornish demonstrated, albeit in a small group of patients, a slight but significant reversal of cardiac disease without any drugs or surgery. His program involved a ten-per-cent-fat vegetarian diet, a supervised exercise program, meditation and counselling.

The problem with Ornish's study is the difficulty in deciding the contribution from each component of the trial. Was it the diet, the exercise or the improved coping skills from the stress-management techniques that reversed the disease?

Another major issue is that it is not real-world stuff. The diet is bland and uninteresting, and would probably last about a week for most people. This type of diet is almost impossible to follow.

THE ZONE DIET

This diet is very similar to the South Beach diet, focusing on the benefits especially in those people with insulin resistance or who have even progressed to diabetes. The Zone diet was made popular by Dr Barry Sears.

THE WEIGHT WATCHERS DIET

The traditional Weight Watchers diet focuses on low-fat foods and portion sizes. Complementing this is a points system to maintain motivation and monitor the success of the program.

The diet debate will probably never be concluded satisfactorily. In my view, the best diet for maintenance of good health lies somewhere in the middle of the extremes. Trying to achieve a balance in our diet should be part of our normal life strategies, just as we should try to achieve balance in all aspects of living. It is my opinion that Atkins' and Ornish's diets are imbalanced, as they expect people to go to extremes rather than to live a moderate life. The Zone and Weight Watchers programs are more moderate, lying closer to the middle and are easier to follow.

In the study of the four diets mentioned earlier in the chapter, the most successful dieters were those who saw their program through to its completion. The bottom line here is very straightforward. Diets are effective and are of benefit if you put in the hard work, but most people are not prepared to do so. Studies have shown that anyone involved in a diet or weight-loss program has only a three per cent chance of continuing to lose weight in the third year after commencing the program. Why? Because they don't stick to it!

We humans are a funny lot. We put faith in the most bizarre notions, including magic pills that burn fat and machines that, when applied for a few minutes every day, will give us a flat stomach. Many people will allow a surgeon to perform a mutilating gastric procedure – anything but make lifestyle changes. The reality is that for most people, diets don't work. We go on diets like we go on a holiday. Few people can take a permanent holiday nor follow a permanent diet.

Occasionally, however, we do see people who have achieved and sustained dramatic weight loss. This is done through attitudinal shifts and lifestyle changes. Diets don't work for two main reasons. Firstly, the first month or so of following any diet usually sees a significant weight loss of around 3–5kg. This weight loss is usually in the form of water and muscle.

It takes up to six months of persistent dieting to mobilise those more ingrained fat stores, i.e. the weight you really want to lose. Thus, after you have lost the initial 3–5kg, you seem to have reached a plateau and after no further success on the program, you tend to slip back to your old habits. The problem is, you don't put back the initial water and muscle lost; you replace this with fat. So, each time you diet, you become flabbier.

The second and most important reason why diets don't work is the lack of a lifelong commitment. If you are truly serious about achieving all the points outlined in Chapter 6, you must see the Walker Lifestyle Program as a long-term undertaking.

Twelve-week programs, diet pills and magic potions to 'blast your fat' don't work. What works is motivation, discipline and a lifelong commitment.

CHAPTER 8

Body type origins

Despite the constant messages from conventional health professionals over the past 20 to 30 years regarding the value of the low-fat, high-carbohydrate diet as the most appropriate way to eat for the entire population, it is obvious that what works for one person doesn't always work for the next.

Why do some people enjoy savoury foods, whilst others prefer sweet? Why are some people constantly hungry or 'obsessed with food', whilst others forget to eat? Why do some people crave exercise, whilst others need a gun to their head before they move? Why are some people tall and skinny, whilst others are short and fat? The answer to all of these questions is that we're all different. So it is vital (if the population is to reverse its modern disease trends) that we individualise our health advice and reject the 'one size fits all' diets, exercise programs, and stress-management concepts.

Why are we different? Because our prehistoric ancestors evolved in different places. The most important determinant of our bodily characteristics, ideal diet, exercise capacities and even aspects of our personalities is the environment in which our ancestors lived. Environmental stimuli such as climate, available food, ratio of daylight to darkness, and cultural habits have set the foundation for our inherent metabolisms. So the same type of diet cannot work for everybody. Many nutrition experts point to the Inuit or the Hunzas from Pakistan as examples of modern populations that do not experience atherosclerosis or its resulting diseases. They claim that these people's diets and lifestyles must protect them against modern Western illnesses.

I believe that a person's prehistoric ancestors' place of evolution has a strong influence over their dietary predilections, body type and exercise preferences.

THE INUIT

As a race, the Inuit make a fascinating study. They are the natives of Alaska and the sparsely populated Arctic circle. Their ancestors lived and evolved in an environment that was cold, lacked vegetation and was difficult to travel through.

The traditional Inuit diet is full of fat, consisting of seal and walrus, with seal oil used as a dipping sauce.

Other meats include caribou, reindeer, moose, geese, ducks and quail-like birds. Of course, there is also a wide variety of fish and whale meat. The short summers experienced by the Inuit mean that fruit and vegetables are scarce but, when available, include wild blueberries, crowberries and salmon berries.

Over thousands of years the Inuit have evolved to tolerate this diet. The fish provides protein, whale blubber regulates their bowels, and organ meats supply essential vitamins. (Strangely, Inuit restaurants have not taken off in the West!) The Inuit have developed rapid metabolisms which allow them to use fat as their primary fuel, and short intestines for the fast burning of nutrients. Their intestines also have the advantage of reducing the absorption of any extra high-fat, high-protein animal products once the body's needs have been satisfied. Their diet has allowed them to develop an extra fat layer of insulation against the cold.

But nutrition isn't the only difference between the Inuit and people in the West; other aspects of lifestyle are also distinct. The Inuit live in igloos and find it quite difficult to open a garage door. This is not because snow constantly blocks the automatic mechanism – it's because they don't have garage doors! There's not much point having a garage if you don't own a car. On the other hand, cross-country skiing – one of the most taxing and energy-expending forms of exercise there is – is like a 'walk in the park' for the Inuit, as they have evolved a bulky, muscular physique that suits this activity. Manoeuvring through snow and ice by any means is an arduous task, and requires a fit body. It certainly uses up the fat stores. So the Inuit burn off many more calories than an average Western citizen.

Since there are so many differences between the traditional Inuit and modern Western societies in diet, physiology and exercise, it is difficult to know the exact reason for the Inuit's lack of Western disease. But the Inuit's traditional eating and living patterns are diminishing as Western society infiltrates their homes. And as the Inuit adopt a more Western style of living, their rates of obesity, diabetes and cardiovascular disease are increasing. Before Western society influenced the Inuit way of life, the communities often experienced periods of near starvation towards the end of winter, as food became scarce. Like hunter-gatherer communities, the Inuit had to store extra fat in their bodies for these times of famine. This ability to store fat and a Western-style diet laced with trans fats and carbohydrates could be factors in the emergence of cardiovascular disease, with the arrival of Western society.

The Inuit and nutrition

The biochemist Howard Raper once said, 'There are no essential foods – only essential nutrients'. This statement recognised that although there are baseline nutritional requirements for all human beings, below which diseases will occur because of nutrient deficiency, those nutrients can be sourced from a variety of foods, depending on what is available.

I believe that the amount of each nutrient needed (above the base requirement) differs between human races. In my view, the varying metabolisms of humans are the reason for all the controversy over diet and supplementation. Metabolisms differ because of the variations in climate and culture around the world. Much of the Inuit's food, for example, could not be consumed by people used to a Western diet. They would either be sick or find the food completely unpalatable. Humans have evolved so that they can survive on the food available to them in their specific habitat.

How does the Inuit metabolism tolerate such a high-fat, low-carbohydrate diet? To understand this we must be aware of why we eat in the first place.

Carbohydrates and fat are our major fuels, with protein used as a back-up if necessary. The body has a fuel hierarchy based on convenience. It is easier to break down carbohydrates into glucose, so this is usually the primary fuel. If the body is low in carbohydrates then it burns fat as the secondary fuel, but it requires more energy to do so. If neither carbohydrate nor fat is available, then proteins (which are usually the building blocks of cells and enzymes) are converted into glucose, a complex process that occurs in the liver and puts a strain on the kidneys.

The Inuit, who have a habitat where there are few carbohydrates, have large livers and urine volumes to cope with the fat and protein metabolism. (The protein breakdown creates more urea, making the need for higher urine volumes.) When the Inuit have abundant food, their dietary needs are met through their high-fat, low-carbohydrate food, and the fat does not build up in their blood vessel walls, thus avoiding atherosclerosis. The fat doesn't cause health problems in the Inuit because it is the correct type of fat, which is actually protective to the body. Most of the Inuit obtain over 50 per cent of their calorie intake from fat, but have about half the death rate of Canadians or Americans from cardiovascular disease. This natural fat is so vital to the Inuit diet, in fact, that without it, their health deteriorates dramatically. In harsh winter conditions, the animals that are the Inuit's food source lose their fat stores, meaning that the Inuit are forced to eat animals that are fat-depleted, despite still being high in protein. This leads to marked weight loss, rapid muscle breakdown, premature aging and death.

PEOPLE IN HOT CLIMATES

Hot, tropical climates with distinct dry and wet seasons typically have abundant vegetation. The metabolism of the people who evolved in these areas is geared to the fruit and vegetables available. Because it is too hot to be expending a significant amount of energy chasing animals all day, the inhabitants of these regions adapted to be able to use complex carbohydrates as their primary source of fuel.

People living in hot climates have long intestines, which enable them to maximise the absorption of carbohydrates because of their 'slow-burning' metabolism. Consider the Kalahari bushmen. These guys with their sleek bodies, dark skin and rapid metabolisms were built for speed. Their diet is mainly vegetarian. When man first moved from the dense jungles of Central Africa to the open savanna, the food supply changed from softer fruits to a more seed- and grain-based diet. The vegetable/animal consumption of these bushmen – and, for that matter, the Australian Aborigines still existing in a more tribal situation in outback Australia – is in a ratio of 80:20.

What I'm trying to say here is really quite straightforward. Living beings are resilient creatures who either adjust to their environment or die off. The problem with our modern world is that, with the increasing cultural and genetic mix along with our modern reliance on synthetic, processed food, we are eating both the wrong types of food for our particular body types and, in most cases, far too much of it.

THE OKINAWANS

Only one in 10,000 humans will live beyond the age of 100. But on the Japanese island of Okinawa, the rate of centenarians is three times this average, and their rate of all modern diseases in people above 100 years old is extremely low.

Longevity has some genetic basis, but over the past 40 to 50 years we have seen a significant increase in longevity in developed countries, which is felt to be due to improved disease treatment and greater emphasis on preventative strategies. The Okinawans have a strong genetic tendency towards longevity and access to modern medicine – the combination makes them the longest living people on the planet. They exist in a lush, subtropical archipelago and consume the natural diet offered by their environment.

Okinawans have a body mass which is below the average of most modern societies. In the United States, over 60 per cent of the adult population has a body mass index greater than 26; the Okinanwans' average is between 20 and 22. Their diet contains a significant amount of low glycemic index (GI) carbohydrates. They practice a mild form of calorie restriction known as Hara Hachi Bu, which means they consume around 10 per cent fewer calories than would generally be recommended for their body size.

Other Okinawan lifestyle factors are also important when considering their longevity rates. They are regular exercisers and, unlike many other Japanese, have a low rate of smoking. Alcohol is consumed in moderation. Their stress levels and coping mechanisms are excellent, helped by their living in an isolated, caring community where older people are respected and not placed in aged-care facilities.

Interestingly the younger Okinawans who are not following their traditional lifestyle are adopting a more Western way of living, gaining weight and smoking more. Their rate of heart disease is moving closer to that seen in other developed countries. And when a group of Okinawans moved to Brazil, their life expectancy became 17 years less than those who remained in their native region.

OTHER WORLD COMMUNITIES

FINLAND

In the 1960s and 1970s, the Fins had the highest rate of heart disease in the world, closely followed by the Scots. A study in the early 1970s showed the rate of heart disease deaths in Finland was a staggering 700 deaths per 10,000. At that stage the Finnish diet was centred on pork and dairy products. The Fins were not overweight, but they did have a high rate of smoking.

The Finnish Government encouraged the population to adopt a healthier lifestyle, with an increased consumption of fruit and vegetables and cessation of smoking. By the mid-1990s, the Fins' rate of heart disease had halved.

Israel

In Israel, fat consumption is much lower than in the United States, but strangely the rates of heart disease, obesity, common cancers and diabetes are higher. I believe that though there may be some genetic factors involved, a major reason is the Israeli diet, which includes an excessive amount of Omega 6 fats in the form of safflower, sunflower, corn and soy bean oil. It is also interesting to note that the diet has a relatively low intake of animal fat.

Some commentators suggest that the Israelis' disease rates are related to the stress of being in the middle of the Arab–Israeli tensions. But if this were so, I would expect the same disease rates to be present in the Arabs; instead, Arabs from the same region have much less disease and eat differently. For one thing, they consume a great deal of extra virgin olive oil.

CHAPTER 9

Introduction to body types

How do we stay healthy? How do we keep fit? How do we avoid weight gain? What is the best way to manage stress? How do we avoid succumbing to a major disease? I believe that the answers to all these important questions are different for each person. So often we hear one scientific study promising benefits from a diet, drug or surgical procedure, only for it to be refuted by another study. This, in my view, is because of the differences between the people being studied, rather than one of the studies being wrong.

Although our bodies have evolved to the point where we can distinguish ourselves from other animals, we certainly come in many different shapes, sizes and colours.

For that reason we need individual programs suited to our own unique body design.

For too long, modern medicine has adopted the 'one size fits all' approach, which is obviously not working. I believe it is time to abandon quick-fix medicine, and to return to each person the responsibility of their health and wellbeing. Whilst we strive to maintain the place of the individual in most other aspects of life, we are happy for modern medicine to develop pharmaceutical agents, surgical procedures and other interventions without catering for individual variations.

GENETICS

There is a new speciality emerging in medicine that will hopefully bring about the ability to cater for individuals more successfully: the field of genetics. Although there is a basic set of genetic requirements to satisfy the definition of a human being, there are also enormous variations within the human genome (the 'map' of typical human DNA) that allow us to be individuals. The variations affect our external appearance as well as our different responses to the environment we live in, including food, drink, drugs, poisons and even climate. The mapping of the human genome will soon allow doctors to assess an individual's risk of disease, and their likely response to drugs and diet.

How can recognising that differences exist between humans help us to live and eat healthily? First we must understand the differences, and to do this we have to group together people with similar characteristics.

For centuries, ancient wisdom from India and China has been used to recognise different body types, and certain medical practices have arisen based on them. Ayurvedic medicine, originating from India, presents three main body types known as doshas. Based on the dominance of one of these doshas, specific dietary, herbal, exercise and other suggestions are said to restore health balance.

A chiropractor, Dr William Sheldon, suggested three specific body types for men and a further fourth type for women. There appears to be a correlation between these types and the Ayurvedic doshas. There has also been further refinement of these types by Dr Elliot Abravanel to correspond with glandular organs within the body.

At this juncture, I would like to make a few important points about the entire concept of body typing, especially pertaining to the 'dominant gland' theory.

The aim of this book is to show how 'diets don't work'. What works is a lifelong commitment to maintaining a healthy lifestyle program. We all need to achieve ideal body weight by reducing our calorie intake and increasing our activity. Thus, the 'calories in' versus the 'calories burnt' concept is more important than the concept of body typing. However, after you have achieved the ideal body weight, then you can further refine your health, energy levels and general feeling of well-being by introducing principles of the body typing program.

Let me also state that the body typing *principles* have been around for many years and are certainly not my original work. I do, however, believe they are important 'fine-tuning' additions to the Dr Walker Lifestyle Program.

You will not find 'body typing' in any medical textbook.

It has not been studied in long-term clinical trials, and for those of you who rely purely on 'evidence-based medicine', I'd suggest you skip this section and follow the basic principles of the Dr Walker Lifestyle Program.

I must, however, state that I have been developing individualised programs in my own practice for the past twenty years, and have found that a body-typing approach works for the majority of people.

Furthermore, the 'dominant gland theory' is just that – a theory. But, it is the most logical explanation for how and why body typing works. When you examine the menus towards the end of this book, you will see definite differences between the proposed types, but all the food is healthy, regardless of your body type.

Whichever system of body typing we choose, the basic principles are the same: we each have a dominant dosha, embryonic or genetically determined body type, or gland, which exerts the most influence on our body.

THE DOMINANT GLAND SYSTEM

For this book, I am using the dominant gland system of body typing. There are four main glandular regions of the body: the controller (pituitary), thyroid, adrenal and gonadal glands.

The theory is that we are all genetically primed to have one of our glands as dominant. Subtle differences in our genetic make-up determine which is our dominant gland, and this has a profound effect on our body shape, fat distribution, energy levels, preferred food, clothing and weather, and on many other aspects of our lives. Our dominant gland determines our metabolic function, energy use and the use of micronutrients.

Metabolic function

Different glands are active during different times of the day. It has been known for many years that the body's metabolic functions vary according to the circadian rhythm (the cyclical secretion of hormones throughout the day). It is important to eat most of our day's food during our dominant gland's most active time, as this is when the body does much of its fat burning. Eating during our dominant gland's 'down time' leads to weight gain and a feeling of sluggishness.

It is also important to eat foods that are more stimulatory to the non-dominant glands, as eating foods that stimulate the dominant gland will lead to it secreting too much of its hormone and, over time, the dominant gland will wear out. The difficulty is that eating foods that stimulate our dominant gland makes us feel good, and we tend to crave these foods. We all enjoy the endorphin release experienced when we consume our favourite foods. But this dominant gland stimulation gives us an acute burst of energy and wellbeing which is followed by an energy crash afterwards.

(This is an identical situation to drug abuse. Use of drugs such as ecstasy or cocaine induces the acute release of dopamine, which leads to a feeling of pleasure. However, the drugs over-release stored dopamine and once they have worn off, there is no further dopamine to maintain the feeling of wellbeing. The crash, whether it be from ecstasy, cocaine or the wrong food, does not feel good.)

As a general rule the glands above the waist (controller and thyroid) are more active during the morning, and the glands below the waist (adrenal and gonads) are more active between mid-afternoon and evening.

Energy use and nutrient intake will be discussed within each body type chapter.

Dominant glands and stress

Stress is defined as a great pressure or strain, and it can overwhelm any body type. Stress over-stimulates the dominant gland by releasing the gland's hormones, thereby depleting the body's reserves of these hormones.

If not rectified, this situation can lead to tiredness and cravings, usually for the food that stimulates the dominant gland, which, if given in to, will lead to further over-stimulation of the gland. This produces a vicious cycle which, if not interrupted, will cause the dominant gland to fail, leading to weight gain. The weight gain results from the excessive consumption of craved foods and the imbalance created by the energy wasted in having to metabolise these foodstuffs.

DISCOVERING YOUR DOMINANT GLAND

How can we make use of the information about dominant glands? In the following chapters, each of the body types is considered in detail, with programs giving advice on how to eat and live in the healthiest way according to body type. For these chapters to be of any use, it is first important to decide where we fit in to the four body types. Then it is important to learn and adopt the best methods of achieving balance for our type. Vital questions to ask are:

- What is my dominant gland?
- What factors lead to over-stimulation of that gland?
- How can I restore balance to my system?

Each of these questions will be addressed in the following chapters.

It is important to realise that not everyone will derive enormous benefits from the body type programs. It is very difficult to overcome many years of learnt bad behaviours and metabolic priming. However, regardless of your age, following your body type program as closely as you can will make you feel better and reduce your risk of certain diseases.

One of the most comprehensive studies of the body type subject was performed by Dr Elliot Abravanel in his book *Dr Abravanel's Body Type Diet and Lifetime Nutrition Plan*. He points out that it is not always possible to be sure of your body type, and suggests that around 35 per cent of people fit clearly within one body type, 40 per cent have some characteristics but not all, while the remaining 25 per cent do not appear to fit into any particular group. Dr Abravanel believes that the reason why a quarter of people are difficult to fit in to any one type may be due to one of the following five factors.

- The person is following an excellent diet for their type and all four glandular regions are working well.
- The person may be more than 15 kilograms overweight.
- Certain genetic backgrounds have characteristics more suited to their racial origin than their body type.
- The modern era has seen the advent of cosmetic surgery. If you don't like your appearance, pay someone to change it.
- Once a person has matured beyond 50 years and their inherent sex hormone status has changed, so may their shape and physiology.

So, at best, we are trying to achieve the closest possible fit when deciding which body type we are.

BOAST CHARACTERISTICS

The BOAST system helps us to determine a person's body type. It is based on a series of body characteristics: Breast size; Obesity (ease in gaining weight and fat distribution); Arm, leg and hand size; Skull and face size and shape; and Trunk size. Additional features such as cravings, energy levels, and exercise and weather preferences can also assist in the process of identifying a body type.

The table below gives an overview of the BOAST characteristics. Try to decide which description for each characteristic suits you. This will give you an idea of whether you are a definite body type or a mix. If most of your 'best fit' descriptions are found in one body type column, you have found your dominant gland and body type.

	Body types			
	Controller	**Thyroid**	**Adrenal**	**Gonadal**
Breast size	+ +	+	+ + +	+ – + +
Obesity	Weight gained easily. Generalised distribution, but particularly abdominal.	Difficult to gain weight. Distributed below waist/ upper hips.	Weight gained easily. Distributed on trunk.	Weight gained easily. Distributed on hips, outer thighs, buttocks.
Arms/legs	Short limbs	Long limbs	Proportioned. Square hands, sturdy fingers.	Small, tapering hands.
Skull/head	Large, youthful face. Round head.	Sharp, small head.	Round face.	Oval/ heart-shaped face.
Trunk	Rectangular.	Long, thin trunk.	Shoulders wider than hips.	Hips wider than shoulders.

The following sections give more in-depth descriptions of the BOAST characteristics as well as the additional features of each body type. They will enable you either to confirm your body type, or to decide which one you are if it hasn't been immediately clear.

Once you have identified and read about your 'best fit' body type here, you can then turn to your specific body type chapter, which sets out your program for optimum health.

It will also be useful to read about the other body types, as you may have certain characteristics that are found predominantly in another type. And it may help you to better understand the people around you!

THE CONTROLLER BODY TYPE

CONTROLLER TYPE CHARACTERISTICS

BREASTS – Controller type females usually have medium-sized breasts.

OBESITY – It is not difficult for an out-of-balance Controller type to gain generalised weight. Abdominal obesity is common, with a strong propensity to insulin resistance.

ARMS/LEGS – Controller types may be either quite short or quite tall – it is less common for them to be somewhere in the middle. The short Controller types tend to have limbs that are short in relation to their trunk.

SKULL/HEAD – Controller types tend to have a rounded head with a large, youthful face. Others often make the comment that they look younger than their age.

TRUNK – The Controller type's trunk appears rectangular in appearance.

CONTROLLER TYPE ADDITIONAL FEATURES

Active time This type's dominant gland is most active during the morning period.

Cravings The classic Controller type loves and craves dairy products. Ice cream, yoghurt, milk and cheese would usually be the first choice for this type.

Weather Give a Controller type a tropical paradise rather a skiing holiday. This type doesn't like the cold, and tends to 'feel' the cold as well.

Energy Controller types have most energy in the morning. There is some waning of energy in the afternoon, but if Controller types follow the correct program, they can maintain excellent energy levels throughout the day.

Personality Of all the types, the Controller tends to be the most introverted. They are typically detached thinkers, analytical, and ideas-oriented.

Wellbeing The Controller is probably the most self-sufficient of all the types. They are able to enjoy their own company and like quiet time alone, engaged in activities such as meditation and walking.

THE THYROID BODY TYPE

THYROID TYPE CHARACTERISTICS

BREASTS – Thyroid type females have small breasts, complementing their slender figure.

OBESITY – Of all the groups, the Thyroid type has the most difficulty gaining weight. When they do, it becomes a spare tyre, just below the waist and at the upper part of the hips.

Thyroid types (usually up until menopause for females and andropause – the decline in testosterone between the ages of 45–55 years – for males) appear to be able to eat what they like without significant weight gain. This is because they have very efficient metabolisms.

ARMS/LEGS – Long limbs in proportion to a long trunk is characteristic of the Thyroid type.

SKULL/HEAD – Thyroid types have a sharp, small, pointed head.

TRUNK – A long, thin trunk is complemented by a narrow front–back diameter (i.e., if you are narrow from the middle of the breastbone to your thoracic spine, you have a narrow front–back diameter).

THYROID TYPE ADDITIONAL FEATURES

Active time This type's dominant gland is most active during the morning period.

Cravings Thyroid types will head straight to the carbohydrates – give them pasta, bread and sweets any day, as opposed to meats and spices.

Weather Thyroid types like hot, humid and bright weather. Being 'all skin and bones' means that they dislike dry, windy and cold weather.

Energy Thyroid types can perform at what seems like a frenetic pace for a while but then they crash. They are the people who (for no apparent reason) have to spend a day resting because they are so exhausted. People who are not Thyroid types find it difficult to comprehend this level of exhaustion.

Personality This type talks quickly, is anxious and quite unpredictable. They have a tendency to be moody.
Wellbeing At times, peace and contentment are difficult to achieve for the Thyroid type. With their moody, variable states of mind, it doesn't take much for them to plunge into either a period of fatigue or a need to withdraw from other people. A balanced, disciplined lifestyle program will offer the best chance of stable moods.

THE ADRENAL BODY TYPE

ADRENAL TYPE CHARACTERISTICS

BREASTS – Adrenal type females tend to have large breasts with small hips and bottom. The breasts become even larger with weight gain. When the Adrenal type male gains weight, a significant amount of fat is deposited around his chest.
OBESITY – It is not difficult for Adrenal types to gain weight. When this happens it is usually confined to the trunk region, with fat folds around the back, and a fat chest and abdomen, but without much gain around the arms and legs.
ARMS/LEGS – Adrenal types are of average height with equally proportioned arms and legs. Their hands are square and they have sturdy fingers.
SKULL/FACE – The Adrenal type has a round face and an average-sized head.
TRUNK – The trunk of an Adrenal type is like an upside-down triangle. They tend to have broad shoulders tapering down to a narrow waist and small hips.

Adrenal type additional features

Active time This type's dominant gland is most active during the late afternoon to early evening.

Cravings Adrenal types tend to bypass the sweet stuff and go straight for the savouries. This type likes to have a solid, hot meal every day.

Exercise This type is geared for action. Having a switched-on sympathetic nervous system (the fear-flight-fight system) means they are like warriors: their well-developed muscular system ensures rapid action and motion when any danger arises.

Weather Most Adrenal types like cold weather. Their dominant adrenal gland means that they generate a lot of internal heat, so the last thing they need is to be even hotter.

Energy Adrenal types usually have a constant supply of energy as long as they can maintain reasonable balance in their bodies. It takes significant imbalance to make Adrenal types have an energy crash.

Personality Adrenal types are often strong, driven people with initiative and willpower. Although they are able to display great enthusiasm, joy and laughter, the downside is obsessive competitiveness with a proneness to anger and hostility. The excessively driven perfectionist who flies off the handle when things go wrong is characteristic of a more negative Adrenal type.

THE GONADAL BODY TYPE

GONADAL TYPE CHARACTERISTICS

Around 50 per cent of females fit into the typical Gonadal body type.

BREASTS The Gonadal type can have small to slightly above average-sized breasts.

OBESITY Gonadal types find it easy to gain weight, which will be distributed on the buttocks and outer thighs.

ARMS/LEGS This type has small hands with tapering fingers. Their arms and legs tend to be average in length, with larger upper thighs.

SKULL/HEAD The Gonadal type's head is oval or heart-shaped.

TRUNK The trunk of a Gonadal type resembles a triangle with the tip pointing up. They tend to have wide hips and narrow shoulders.

GONADAL TYPE ADDITIONAL FEATURES

Active time This type's dominant gland is most active during the afternoon and evening.

Cravings Creamy and spicy foods, and heavy organ meats (brains, liver, kidneys) are the prominent cravings for the Gonadal type.

Exercise The Gonadal type tends to be quite athletic and typically seeks and enjoys exercise.

Weather For the Gonadal type weather preferences are not clear-cut, and often depend on the helper function.

Some Gonadal types prefer cooler weather, but this is not always the case.

Energy Although appearing to have boundless energy and always ready to give of herself (especially for those whom she loves), the Gonadal type is prone to sudden bursts of fatigue. Gonadal types are usually strong, both emotionally and physically, but occasionally some time out is necessary. Gonadal types tend to have greater energy in the latter part of the day, so if there is an imbalance this increased energy from mid-afternoon to evening is lost.

Personality Gonadal types are warm, outgoing and people-oriented. They are compassionate, caring, nurturing types.

Now that you have understood the reasons why diets don't work, and how our modern world has contributed to the majority of our major, modern illnesses, it is time to make a commitment to following a lifelong program that will work.

If you follow the Walker Lifestyle program, you will achieve your ideal body, gain energy and develop a greater sense of well-being.

PART 3

THE DR WALKER LIFESTYLE PROGRAM

CHAPTER 10

The Controller body type

The controller, or pituitary, is a vitally important little gland that sits at the base of the brain and is the conductor in the hormonal orchestra. It directs the entire flow and concentration of hormones through the body. The gland is under the control of a specialised area in the brain known as the hypothalamus. Small peptides (a few amino acids joined together) known as neuro-transmitters are released by the hypothalamus when it receives messages and stimuli from both within and without the body, such as fluid status, hunger, eating, sexual stimulation and satisfaction. The controller then sends hormones throughout the body based on the messages. The messages arrive incessantly, so the controller is in a constant state of flux.

HORMONES PRODUCED BY THE CONTROLLER GLAND

Before adulthood, the controller regulates growth by secreting growth hormone to the body. Once growing has stopped, the growth hormone still has effects on the body in maintaining blood pressure and connective tissue integrity. It is believed by some that growth hormone has anti-aging properties, and many people are paying big money for treatments with the hormone in the form of injections, pills or nasal sprays.

The controller also regulates the sex hormones secreted by the ovaries in women and the testes in men. The female sex hormones, oestrogen and progesterone, determine many aspects of female body shape, sex drive and menstruation, not to mention their vital role in the preparation and maintenance of pregnancy. The male sex hormone, testosterone, with its intricate relationship to muscle growth and bulk, influences male body shape, maintains libido and governs some of the more aggressive aspects of male behaviour.

Two other important hormones are released by the controller, which are vital in the regulation of weight: adrenocorticotrophic hormone (ACTH), which directs the release of cortisone by the adrenal glands (cortisone helps with the maintenance of normal cellular function and fluid status) and thyroid-stimulating hormone (TSH), which instructs the thyroid to release thyroxine (the active hormone) which, in turn, sets the metabolic rate of cells.

Hormonal secretion throughout the body is cyclic rather than constant. Secretion cycles can be daily (diurnal variation) or, in the case of female sex hormones, spread throughout the month. Any type of external or internal stress, from appetite (both for food and sex) to temperature perception and even mood, can cause variations in this cyclical secretion. The variations partly explain why humans are so changeable – for example, why we sometimes have lots of energy whilst at other times are fatigued. The variations in all our bodily activities have a strong relationship to this cyclical nature of hormone secretion.

Over-stimulation of the controller gland by these variations can cause a general mis-regulation of all the glandular systems in the body, leading to subtle glandular hypofunction.

THE CONTROLLER TYPE AND DISEASE

Many types of disease can affect the controller gland, causing it to over- or under-perform. The gland is prone to tumour formation (probably because it is so active). Although the tumours are usually benign, they can have disastrous consequences on the body, depending on the type of hormone-secreting cell that forms the tumour, and the local effects on the brain from the tumour's growth.

Probably the most common tumour of the controller gland is the prolactinoma. Prolactin is the hormone released soon after birth that induces milk formation in the breast. It also interacts with other brain chemicals in lactating women and, depending on the nature of this interaction, may lead to feelings of either contentment or post-natal depression. A person with a prolactinoma often gains an enormous amount of weight (accumulating all over the body) and may suffer from a condition known as galactorrhoea (milk discharged from the breast in a non-lactating female). This can also lead to cessation of menstruation.

Tall Controller types have a tendency towards ectomorphic forms of disease, such as chronic musculoskeletal disorders, valvular heart disease and, at a more serious level, arterial rupture. They may also suffer from anxiety and, to a lesser extent, depression. The shorter Controller types are more prone to diabetes and insulin resistance, and their related problems.

THE CONTROLLER TYPE AND STRESS

There is no doubt that stress affects the entire body, but its manifestations are vastly different between individuals. From a metabolic viewpoint, chronic stress in a Controller type (such as problems at work or home) leads to over-stimulation throughout the glandular system, until all the glands are exhausted.

The main stimulants of the controller gland are dairy products, which release prolactin, the hormone released during breast-feeding, which induces a feeling of contentment. So when Controller types are stressed, they crave dairy products, as the release of prolactin gives partial relief from the stressful feelings. Unfortunately this relief is only short-lived, and more dairy is then necessary. If large quantities of dairy are eaten by Controller types, their dominant gland will become further overstimulated.

CASE STUDY: CONTROLLER BODY TYPE

Scott is a 51-year-old software consultant. He is 1.59 metres tall, but weighs an unhealthy 85 kilograms, making him obese. (He loves ice cream and eats it every day.) His weight distribution is general, including puffy hands, stodgy fingers, and thick, puffy ankles and feet. Despite his weight gain, he still has a youthful appearance. He has a rounded head.

When he was younger, Scott's parents consulted an endocrinologist (a speclialist in glandular disorders), as Scott appeared to be a late maturer and didn't grow through his late teens. No specific abnormalities were found during this assessment, and Scott's parents were reassured that he was simply short of stature.

Scott has always been self-conscious about his height and, possibly as a consequence of this, prefers his own company. He married in his mid-thirties, but this relationship only lasted for a few years; he has been single since then. He works in the computer industry, and his main interests are watching movies and playing on his computer. He lives in Brisbane, and travels to northern Queensland each year for a fishing holiday with some friends.

He has been diagnosed with late-onset diabetes, and has suffered two bouts of severe chest pain, but on both occasions his stress test was normal so no further action was taken.

Scott is a classic Controller type who needs an immediate change in his life habits. He should avoid dairy products and adopt a more protein-based diet. He should commence an exercise program and have a more thorough evaluation for cardiovascular disease.

Cases like Scott's are common, and are 'heart attacks waiting to happen'. The diagnosis of diabetes carries with it the same prognosis as established stable heart disease, and requires aggressive risk-factor modification to prevent one of the more serious complications of heart disease such as heart attack, stroke or sudden cardiac death.

THE CONTROLLER TYPE LIFESTYLE PROGRAM

EXERCISE

As they have a slight frame, Controller types do well with weight training. Their bodies are usually very flexible. The best program for the Controller type is a regular aerobic program with equal concentration on isometric exercises and other forms of resistance training.

FOODS TO EAT REGULARLY

- Vegetables, including avocados
- Protein (not dairy) at every meal (including eggs,

organ meats, red meat or chicken, plenty of fish, daily natural nuts)
- Extra virgin olive oil
- Fenugreek herbal tea

These foods stimulate the non-dominant glands and therefore promote a balanced secretion of hormones.

Foods to eat in moderation

- Fruit
- Wholegrains

Although fruits and wholegrains are very healthy, excessive carbohydrates contribute to pituitary stimulation.

Foods to minimise

- Dairy products
- Caffeine
- Sugar- and flour-based foods

All of the above foods stimulate the dominant gland of Controller types.

Eating principles

- Eat more vegetables than fruit.
- Reverse the typical eating order – the Controller type should have a substantial breakfast, a reasonable lunch and a light dinner. This is sometimes difficult to achieve, but should be followed most of the time for your program to be successful.

- Avoid snacking, especially in the late afternoon, when Controller types reach a low ebb. They usually crave ice cream, yoghurt or cheese, and occasionally something sweet or even starchy. This will be a disaster for your program: have an apple or orange if you must eat something. A herbal tea will help to abate the cravings.

SEVEN-DAY FOOD PROGRAM

The following meal plans are suggestions for Controller types to encourage eating within the appropriate food categories. Similar types of recipes with equivalent caloric intake are acceptable within the program. (See Chapter 14 for recipes.)

DAY 1

Breakfast
Dr Walker's super-charged breakfast for C types:
10–15 natural nuts (preferably walnuts, almonds and macadamias)
1–2 dsp LSA (crushed linseeds, sunflower seeds and almonds)
1 heaped dsp unprocessed bran
Combination of blueberries (¼ cup), 2–3 strawberries and ½ banana
150 ml low-fat milk blended with 50–100 g low-fat yoghurt
or

1 fried egg (in small amount of extra virgin olive oil) on 1 piece wholegrain toast
1 glass freshly squeezed juice or 1 cup tea (preferably green or fenugreek)

Lunch
Turkey, cranberry sauce, lettuce and 1 slice low-fat cheese on 2 slices wholegrain bread
1 piece fruit
Herbal tea

Dinner
Cajun chicken (see recipe on page 191)

DAY 2

Breakfast
Combination of ¼ punnet blueberries, 3 strawberries, ½ banana and ½ mango

Lunch
Salad using a variety of vegetables, e.g. lettuce, tomatoes, mushrooms, celery, cucumber, capsicum and olives
1 cup tea (black, green or herbal)

Dinner
Peppered steak, and Greek salad (see recipes on pages 204 and 195)

Day 3

Breakfast

Berry smoothie (see recipe on page 210)
Natural peanut butter on 1 slice wholegrain bread
Herbal tea

Lunch

Smoked salmon, capers and light mayonnaise on 2 slices wholegrain bread
Herbal tea

Dinner

Spicy perch fillets with capsicum and tomato salsa (see recipe on page 213)

Day 4

Breakfast

Dr Walker's super-charged breakfast for C types:
10–15 natural nuts (preferably walnuts, almonds and macadamias)
1–2 dsp LSA (crushed linseeds, sunflower seeds and almonds)
1 heaped dsp unprocessed bran
Combination of blueberries (¼ cup), 2–3 strawberries and ½ banana
150 ml low-fat milk blended with 50–100 g low-fat yoghurt

or

1 boiled egg on 1 piece wholegrain toast
1 glass freshly squeezed juice or 1 cup herbal tea

Lunch
Spinach soup and tofu (see recipe on page 215)
Herbal tea

Dinner
Celery and onion omelette, and stir-fried green beans (see recipes on pages 192 and 218)

Day 5

Breakfast
Corn pancakes (see recipe on page 193)

Lunch
Mashed, hard-boiled egg mixed with yoghurt and curry powder on 2 slices wholegrain bread
Herbal tea

Dinner
Teriyaki lamb stir-fry (see recipe on page 221)

Day 6

Breakfast
Dr Walker's super-charged breakfast for C types:
10–15 natural nuts (preferably walnuts, almonds and macadamias)
1–2 dsp LSA (crushed linseeds, sunflower seeds and almonds)
1 heaped dsp unprocessed bran
Combination of blueberries (¼ cup), 2–3 strawberries and ½ banana

150 ml low-fat milk blended with 50–100 g low-fat yoghurt

Lunch

Slice 1 carrot, 1 stick of celery, 1 avocado, 1 red capsicum and 1 zucchini. Dip vegetables into homemade mayonnaise (see recipe on page 200)

Dinner

Quick-cook salmon or tuna, and Cauliflower Neapolitan (see recipes on pages 206 and 191)

Day 7

Breakfast

Smoked salmon strips with ½ avocado on 1 slice wholegrain toast

Banana smoothie (see recipe on page 210)

Lunch

2 boiled eggs, lettuce and spring onions on 2 slices wholegrain bread

1 apple

Dinner

Lemon chicken stir-fry (see recipe on page 198)

CHAPTER 11

The Thyroid body type

Of all the body types, this is the easiest to pick. Thyroid types are tall and thin, sometimes even gaunt, with long fingers and what looks like more bones than anything else. They may not be the tallest of the tall – often this award goes to the Controller type – but they are usually taller (and definitely skinnier) than most.

The thyroid is a gland that sits at the base of the throat, just below the skin and above the notch of the neck. It is the major regulator of metabolism, and sets the speed at which the cells in the body work by secreting the hormone thyroxine. Excessive thyroxine makes the cells work quickly, whilst reduced thyroxine makes the cells work slowly. An overactive thyroid gland is indicated by a person suffering from weight loss, fast heartbeat, diarrhoea, sweating and anxiety – just as you would expect from a system that is working too fast. An underactive thyroid gland is signified by the opposite – a mentally slow, depressed, tired person with a slow pulse and constipation – a system working too slowly.

The Thyroid type is not suffering from thyroid disease, but as the thyroid is the dominant gland it certainly regulates the system to maximum efficiency. Thus the balanced Thyroid type is wiry, speedy, quick-thinking and energetic. Also, as thyroxine is the major metabolic regulator, having the thyroid as the dominant gland will mean that this type's metabolism works in the upper range of normal.

THE THYROID TYPE AND DISEASE

Although I'm not disputing that the condition chronic fatigue syndrome exists, I do believe that many people diagnosed with this condition are instead out-of-balance Thyroid types.

The type is prone to thyroid failure and other associated endocrine (glandular) disorders. They commonly experience palpitations and muscular chest pain syndromes. Thyroid types also commonly experience gastro-intestinal problems. However, Thyroid types are the least prone to late-onset diabetes.

THE THYROID TYPE AND STRESS

If the Thyroid type over-stimulates their metabolism with the wrong foods, excessive calories, a poor exercise program or a difficult, stressful life, the thyroid gland will cease to function efficiently and at times fail, leading to an under-active thyroid and the need for thyroxine-replacement therapy.

Every aspect of our life determines what we crave, how we behave, our own inherent level of motivation and discipline, and imbalances. Thyroid types should have three regular meals per day, but often they forget to eat. Their eating is variable: occasionally it is voracious, especially when it comes to sweets and carbohydrates, but at other times food is of little interest to them. By ensuring that they eat the correct number of meals each day, Thyroid types can immediately bring part of their life into balance.

CASE STUDY: THYROID BODY TYPE

Margaret is a 61-year-old dance instructor. She has a thin face with rectangular head, and is tall with a long, narrow torso and thin arms and legs. She often craves and consumes pasta and enjoys warm weather.

She has been suffering from palpitations (a sensation of an abnormal heartbeat) over the past few months, along with a progressive feeling of fatigue over many years. She has been troubled since early adulthood by a condition known as inflammatory bowel disease and has required numerous hospitalisations to treat the condition. She has a chronic cough with a runny nose and suffers from recurrent migraine headaches.

Margaret is a classic Thyroid type, has many of the associated diseases and does not eat right for her body type.

Rather than take a holistic approach to Margaret's case, her health professionals have treated each symptom separately. This has led to a situation where Margaret is barely coping, managing multiple ailments and feeling constantly fatigued.

Had she been on a Thyroid body type program from an early age, which includes eating protein at each meal and avoiding carbohydrates, she would have had a much more fulfilling life with fewer ailments. Unfortunately, at the age of 61 her habits and metabolism are so ingrained that, despite commencing the program, she did not experience much improvement, although after a few months she did feel a little better. This case highlights the importance of determining your body type early and following the program.

THE THYROID TYPE LIFESTYLE PROGRAM

Exercise

This type benefits from strength training. They'd be much better lifting weights in the gym than focusing on aerobic activity.

Foods to eat regularly

- Vegetables (5–7 serves per day)
- Protein, including dairy, at every meal (eggs and

organ meats, red meat, chicken, plenty of fish, daily natural nuts)
- Raspberry-based herbal tea

Plant-based foods, especially vegetables, are beneficial and should be encouraged for all groups. Regular protein stimulates the non-dominant glands below the waist, ensuring balanced stimulation.

Foods to eat in moderation

- Fruit (1 piece per day)
- Wholegrains

Although fruits and wholegrains are very healthy, excessive carbohydrates contribute to pituitary stimulation. Excessive fruit can be a strong stimulant of the dominant thyroid gland due to the high fructose content.

Foods to minimise

- Sweets
- Caffeine
- Flour- and sugar-based food

These foods are very stimulatory to the thyroid gland.

Eating principles

- Consume only low GI carbohydrates.
- Balance your meals with close to equal proportions for breakfast, lunch and dinner.
- Avoid snacking, especially with any sugar-based

foods in the late afternoon and evening.
If you must snack, a protein bar, protein shake or even half a hard-boiled egg are preferable.

SEVEN-DAY FOOD PROGRAM

The following meal plans are suggestions for Thyroid types to encourage eating within the appropriate food categories. Similar types of recipes with equivalent caloric intake are acceptable within the program. (See Chapter 14 for recipes.)

DAY 1

Breakfast
Vegetarian omelette (see recipe on page 225)
1 glass freshly squeezed juice or 1 cup herbal tea

Lunch
Leg ham and 1 slice low-fat cheese on 2 slices wholegrain bread, with salad
1 piece fruit

Dinner
Thai beef salad 1 (see recipe on page 222)

DAY 2

Breakfast
Tasty frittata (see recipe on page 220)
Herbal tea

Lunch
Red kidney bean soup (see recipe on page 208)

Dinner
Lemon salmon (see recipe on page 199)

Day 3

Breakfast
Tasty frittata (see recipe on page 220)
Herbal tea
or
Chopped smoked salmon and chives with avocado topping on toast
Herbal tea

Lunch
Spring salad

Dinner
Grilled chicken with tomato salsa (see recipe on page 196)

Day 4

Breakfast
Chop up a large handful of fresh mushrooms (any variety). Fry them in 1 tsp extra virgin olive oil with a selection of vegetables, including chopped shallots or tomatoes. Serve on 1 slice wholegrain toast using avocado as spread.
Herbal tea

Lunch

1 slice low-fat cheese with mustard on 2 slices wholegrain bread, with salad

1 piece fruit

Dinner

Lamb and fennel kebabs, and Avocado and cashew salad (see recipes on pages 197 and 188)

Day 5

Breakfast

Protein boost (see recipe on page 204)

Herbal tea

Lunch

Turkey, cranberry sauce, lettuce and 1 slice low-fat cheese on 2 slices wholegrain bread

1 piece fruit

Dinner

Sesame prawns with asparagus, and Broccoli with almonds (see recipes on pages 209 and 190)

Day 6

Breakfast

Dr Walker's super-charged breakfast for T types:

3–4 dsp walnuts and almonds

1 dsp lecithin

1 dsp LSA (crushed linseeds, sunflower seeds and almonds)
1 dsp unprocessed bran
½ banana and 3 strawberries
150 ml low-fat milk blended with 50–100 g low-fat yoghurt
Herbal tea

Lunch
Greek salad

Dinner
Mexican stuffed chicken, and Steamed greens (see recipes on pages 200 and 216)

Day 7

Breakfast
Banana smoothie (see recipe on page 210)
Smoked salmon strips with ½ avocado on 1 slice wholegrain toast
Herbal tea

Lunch
2 boiled eggs, lettuce and spring onions on 2 slices wholegrain bread
1 apple

Dinner
Fried white fish, and Tofu, lentil and tomato salad (see recipes on pages 194 and 224)

CHAPTER 12

The Adrenal body type

The adrenals are a couple of small triangular glands that sit above the kidneys and, with some contribution from the pancreas, are the dominant glands for this type. They help the body to cope with the various stresses of life by making adrenaline- and cortisone-associated steroid hormones, which are vital for normal body metabolism. As stress and stress hormones are significant drivers in the Adrenal type's body, over-stimulation of the dominant glands will 'wire the Adrenal type for stress'. Adrenaline makes the heart work harder and faster, along with increasing the blood flow to the muscles. This allows the individual to be stronger and react quickly to stress. Cortisone tends to be more involved in sub-acute to chronic stress, mobilising the immune system and allowing the white cells to deal with the stimulus involved.

THE ADRENAL TYPE AND DISEASE

The main Adrenal type diseases are high blood pressure, cardiovascular disease and colon cancer.

The Adrenal type, with driven, perfectionist ways, will strive through one situation to the next trying to live up to their and everyone's expectations, but this behaviour comes at a price. Unless the Adrenal type follows a balanced program, by around the age of 50, distinct problems will emerge.

THE ADRENAL TYPE AND STRESS

It is only logical that someone with the adrenal glands as their dominant system should have a switched on fear-flight-fight system. It is not difficult for an Adrenal type to experience an exaggerated response to stress.

CASE STUDY: ADRENAL BODY TYPE

Mark is a 47-year-old man who has worked all of his life in the building industry. He played first-grade football in his twenties and was a fast, well-built sportsman; he had a very muscular frame at that age. Like any typical Adrenal type, he loves his meat and, like any typical footballer, enjoys his beer. When he retired from football in his early thirties, he continued to exercise until his late thirties and was also working in a physical job on building sites. He is always keen and disciplined but has a bad temper and flies off the handle if things aren't going the way he expected.

He progressed from being a brickie's labourer to being a supervisor, and his work became more administrative than physical. In his early forties, because of an old knee injury, he could no longer perform the same level of exercise and his muscular frame soon turned to fat. He developed significant obesity on his trunk and gained around 20 kilograms over a five-year period.

At the age of 45 he developed severe chest pain and was found to have had a heart attack. A coronary stent was placed in one of the main arteries of his heart, and he remained on statin drugs to lower his cholesterol, and daily aspirin. He was told to lose weight and to cut out fat from his diet, but he was under the mistaken impression that the stent and the drugs would be all he needed.

A few years after the stent was implanted, he began to experience further chest pain and tests showed that he had developed three more severe blockages in his arteries, requiring coronary artery bypass grafting.

Mark is a classic Adrenal type with all of the risk factors and problems that go with it. The advice he was given about starting a low-fat diet was highly appropriate for his body type, but he needed strict guidelines and better explanation for this message to truly sink in. Mark also requires aggressive risk-factor modification. Within six to eight years of the coronary artery bypass grafting the arteries will have become blocked again unless Mark puts greater effort into controlling the factors that caused his disease in the first place.

THE ADRENAL TYPE LIFESTYLE PROGRAM

Exercise

If an Adrenal type spends a lot of time on aerobic exercises (muscle-building work such as weights), they will quickly develop a solid muscular body. However, unless this activity is maintained on a life-long basis, the muscle will rapidly turn to fat.

The best exercise for an Adrenal type (unless they have a strong desire to be a professional body builder) is a combination of aerobic exercise (for example running, swimming), stretching, and Pilates or yoga, with minimal weights, which should be used purely to maintain tone.

Foods to eat regularly

- Fruits and vegetables
- Wholegrain foods including breads, wholegrain pasta and brown rice
- Parsley herbal tea

These foods stimulate the non-dominant glands above the waist, allowing balanced glandular secretion.

Foods to eat in moderation

- Alcohol
- Lower-fat meats such as chicken and turkey
- Nuts
- Caffeine

Although regular, heavy consumption of alcohol (greater

than 3–4 standard glasses of alcohol or cups of coffee) has proven health detriments, evidence has emerged over the past 10–15 years that regular, low dose consumption of alcohol (especially red wine) and coffee (not instant) has some health benefits (see *The Cell Factor*).

As A types tend to be more muscular, they still need a moderate intake of high-quality proteins that have low fat contents.

Foods to minimise

- High-fat foods
- Red and organ meats
- Eggs and shellfish

Excessive stimulation of the adrenal glands with high-fat foods, especially those laden with cholesterol, leads to very easy weight gain. This makes it important for calorie restriction to be the first and most important part of the Adrenal type eating program. Although I am a strong critic of the low-fat diet pushed for years by many elements of the conventional medical and dietary world, the Adrenal type benefits from this type of eating.

Unfortunately, Adrenal types enjoy nothing more than bacon and eggs for breakfast, but this is the worst food for them to eat. This is because the fat in the bacon and the cholesterol in the egg yolk over-stimulate the adrenal glands, leading to excessive cortisol production, a major factor in weight gain. Also, eating this type of meal during the adrenal glands' inactive period (morning to lunch) also over-stimulates glands that would prefer to 'sleep in'.

Eating principles

- Increase your intake of low GI carbohydrates, especially fruits and vegetables. Although this is anathema to you, being a vegetarian is the best way for an Adrenal type to eat.
- The typical eating order for modern society is the best approach for an Adrenal type. Have a small breakfast and lunch and a more substantial evening meal; but don't 'pig out'!
- A piece of fruit is an ideal snack for this type.

SEVEN-DAY FOOD PROGRAM

The following meal plans are suggestions for Adrenal types to encourage eating within the appropriate food categories. Similar types of recipes with equivalent caloric intake are acceptable within the program. (See Chapter 14 for recipes.)

Day 1

Breakfast

Dr Walker's super-charged breakfast for A types:

10–15 natural nuts (preferably walnuts, almonds and macadamias)

1–2 dsp LSA (crushed linseeds, sunflower seeds and almonds)

1 heaped dsp unprocessed bran

Combination of blueberries (¼ cup), 2–3 strawberries and ½ banana

150 ml low-fat milk blended with 50–100 g low-fat yoghurt

or

1 fried or boiled egg on 1 piece wholegrain toast

1 glass freshly squeezed juice or 1 cup herbal tea

Lunch

Asparagus and potato soup (see recipe on page 187)

Dinner

Pasta with broccoli, bacon and chilli (see recipe on page 202)

Day 2

Breakfast

1 bowl rolled oats

1 piece wholegrain toast with Omega 3 margarine

Lunch

2 boiled eggs, lettuce and spring onions on 2 slices wholegrain bread

Dinner

Spicy salmon steak (see recipe on page 214)

Day 3

Breakfast

1 bowl natural muesli with 150 ml low-fat milk

Lunch

1 slice low-fat cheese and mustard on 2 slices wholegrain bread, with salad

Dinner

Chicken burgers, and Stir-fried vegetables (see recipes on pages 193 and 219)

DAY 4

Breakfast

1 piece fruit, any variety

Lunch

Thai beef salad 2 (see recipe on page 222)

Dinner

Spaghetti pomodori (see recipe on page 211)

DAY 5

Breakfast

Dr Walker's super-charged breakfast for A types:

10–15 natural nuts (preferably walnuts, almonds and macadamias)

1–2 dsp LSA (crushed linseeds, sunflower seeds and almonds)

1 heaped dsp unprocessed bran

Combination of blueberries (¼ cup), 2–3 strawberries and ½ banana

150 ml low-fat milk blended with 50–100 g low-fat yoghurt

or
1 fried or boiled egg on 1 piece wholegrain toast
1 glass freshly squeezed juice or 1 cup herbal tea

Lunch
100 g turkey, cranberry sauce, lettuce and 1 slice low-fat cheese on 2 slices wholegrain bread
1 piece fruit

Dinner
Pumpkin soup, and Greek salad (see recipes on pages 206 and 195)

Day 6

Breakfast
1 bowl rolled oats
1 piece wholegrain toast with Omega 3 margarine

Lunch
Greek salad (see recipe on page 195)

Dinner
Provencal fish, and Stir-fried spinach (see recipes on pages 205 and 218)

Day 7

Breakfast
Dr Walker's super-charged breakfast for A types:
10–15 natural nuts (preferably walnuts, almonds and macadamias)

1–2 dsp LSA (crushed linseeds, sunflower seeds and almonds)
1 heaped dsp unprocessed bran
Combination of blueberries (¼ cup), 2–3 strawberries and ½ banana
150 ml low-fat milk blended with 50–100 g low-fat yoghurt
or
1 fried or boiled egg on 1 piece wholegrain toast
1 glass freshly squeezed juice or 1 cup herbal tea

Lunch
Smoked salmon, capers and light mayonnaise on 2 slices wholegrain bread
Herbal tea

Dinner
Nasi Goreng, and Raw vegetable salad (see recipes on pages 201 and 207)

CHAPTER 13

The Gonadal body type

Gonadal types, also known as 'gonadomorphs', are always female, and have their ovaries as the dominant gland. The ovaries are typically dominant in over 50 per cent of the type, whilst the rest have a varying contribution from the other glandular systems as well, which means that some Gonadal types will have characteristics that are normally found in the other types.

THE GONADAL TYPE AND DISEASE

The foods craved by Gonadal types – spicy or creamy foods, and the heavier organ meats – lead to either excess blood flow to the ovaries or increased cholesterol, the basic substrate for steroid hormones, which therefore overworks the gonadal glandular system.

Gonadal type imbalance can also lead to varying gynaecological problems, such as fibroids and ovarian cysts. This type should have regular surveillance for common gynaecological cancers.

THE GONADAL TYPE AND STRESS

As with all body types, stress tends to particularly affect the dominant glandular system. Stress releases adrenaline and cortisone from the adrenal glands. Adrenaline adversely alters blood flow to the ovaries, whereas cortisone affects sex hormone secretion.

THE IMBALANCED GONADAL TYPE

When the Gonadal type is out of balance and starts to gain weight, the weight tends to accumulate in the lower body. This is because the ovaries secrete sex hormones into this area.

SIGNS OF OVER-STIMULATION

Gonadal type imbalance from over-stimulation leads to pelvic congestion and all its consequences. Any factor that over-stimulates the ovaries will lead to an increased release of sex hormones in the buttocks, hips and upper thighs. An over-stimulated Gonadal type will not only gain weight and feel tired, but will also suffer a reduction in sexual desire because of the imbalance.

CASE STUDY: GONADAL BODY TYPE

Adele is a 29-year-old flight attendant with an international airline. She is an attractive young lady with a bubbly personality and has battled with her weight since early childhood. Although she is not typically overweight, she does carry weight around her waist and, to a lesser extent, her hips. She has an olive complexion, is slightly hirsute (has excessive body hair) and is prone to mild acne. Her weight and health deteriorated when she switched from domestic to international flying.

She craves (on a life-long basis) cheese and spicy foods but over the past few years has also relied on sugar hits to maintain her energy after a busy day.

Adele has the full hips of a Gonadal type but also has some of the features of the upper-body glandular systems. This unique combination has led to her current health status. Her periods are regular and very painful. For the past three years she has been diagnosed with polycystic ovarian syndrome. There is a strong association between polycystic ovaries and insulin resistance, explaining the weight gain.

Her full breasts and wide hips combined with her cravings for sweets and rich, spicy foods suggest that she suffers not only from insulin resistance weight gain (abdominal obesity), but also from primary ovarian hyperstimulation, which leads to excessive ovarian blood flow (from the ingestion of rich, spicy foods). This mix of conditions is a recipe for polycystic ovaries. Although drugs have been developed to assist the situation, the first approach should always be a change of lifestyle.

Adele needs to move towards a more balanced high-protein, high-quality fat diet and to avoid synthetic fats, heavier spicy foods and processed carbohydrates. She needs to ensure that three servings of protein are incorporated into her meals per day.

THE GONADAL TYPE LIFESTYLE PROGRAM

EXERCISE

Lower body work increases blood flow and muscle bulk to this area. Weights and resistance training involving the legs, or the use of a rowing machine, should be avoided by Gonadal types. Instead, they should concentrate on aerobic exercise, upper body strength and resistance work, and stretching, using either yoga or Pilates.

FOODS TO EAT REGULARLY

- Fruit and vegetables
- Dairy products (low-fat)
- Low GI carbohydrates
- Fish, chicken, turkey
- Lentils
- Nuts (must be natural – not roasted or salted, and best are walnuts, almonds and macadamias)
- Eggs (evening meal only)

- Tofu (evening meal only)
- Red clover herbal tea

These foods maintain balanced stimulation to the non-dominant glands. In other words, they stimulate the glands above the heart – the controller and thyroid – so balance the stronger output from the ovaries. The Gonadal type will benefit from being mostly vegetarian, as fruits especially have a significant stimulating effect on the thyroid.

Foods to eat in moderation

- Sugar- and caffeine-based drinks (uncarbonated)
- Extra virgin olive oil

Moderate amounts of these foodstuffs will stimulate the non-dominant glands without overstimulating the dominant glands.

Foods to minimise

- Spicy food
- Creamy food
- Red meat

The Gonadal type who craves spicy, creamy foods on a regular basis is certainly out of balance. This type's dominant glands are below the waist and tend to work more in the late afternoon and evening. Thus a combination of creamy and spicy foods, especially for breakfast or lunch, forces the dominant glands to work out of sync and plays havoc with the metabolism. Gonadal types certainly need to follow a regimen that is geared towards low fat.

Eating principles

- Breakfast and lunch should be light, with the main meal eaten at night.
- Snacking is not beneficial for Gonadal types, so if something is needed at these times, fruit and possibly a small helping of nuts would be the best things to eat. Herbal tea, especially consumed during the strongest craving time, is beneficial for the Gonadal type. This will help to reduce food cravings.

SEVEN-DAY FOOD PROGRAM

The following meal plans are suggestions for Adrenal types to encourage eating within the appropriate food categories. Similar types of recipes with equivalent caloric intake are acceptable within the program. (See Chapter 14 for recipes.)

Day 1

Breakfast

Dr Walker's super-charged breakfast for G types:
10–15 natural nuts (preferably walnuts, almonds and macadamias)
1–2 dsp LSA (crushed linseeds, sunflower seeds and almonds)
1 heaped dsp unprocessed bran
Combination of blueberries (¼ cup), 2–3 strawberries and ½ banana

150 ml low-fat milk blended with 50–100 g low-fat yoghurt

or

1 fried or boiled egg on 1 piece wholegrain toast

1 glass freshly squeezed juice or 1 cup herbal tea

Lunch

Baked beans and low-fat cheddar cheese on 2 slices wholegrain bread

Dinner

Avocado pasta, and Greek salad (see recipes on pages 188 and 195)

Day 2

Breakfast

1 bowl rolled oats

1 piece wholegrain toast with Omega 3 margarine

Lunch

Greek salad (see recipe on page 195)

Dinner

Stir-fried chicken, and Tofu, lentil and tomato salad (see recipes on pages 217 and 224)

Day 3

Breakfast

1 bowl natural muesli

Lunch
Mashed hard-boiled egg with natural yoghurt and cracked pepper on 2 slices wholegrain bread

Dinner
Salmon patties, and Special beans (see recipes on pages 209 and 212)

Day 4

Breakfast
1 piece fruit, any variety

Lunch
Lentil soup (see recipe on page 199)

Dinner
Spaghetti with diced tomatoes (see recipe on page 212)

Day 5

Breakfast
Dr Walker's super-charged breakfast for G types:
10–15 natural nuts (preferably walnuts, almonds and macadamias)
1–2 dsp LSA (crushed linseeds, sunflower seeds and almonds)
1 heaped dsp unprocessed bran
Combination of blueberries (¼ cup), 2–3 strawberries and ½ banana
150 ml low-fat milk blended with 50–100 g low-fat yoghurt

or

1 fried or boiled egg on 1 piece wholegrain toast

1 glass freshly squeezed juice or 1 cup herbal tea

Lunch

Raw vegetable salad (see recipe on page 207)

Dinner

Grilled snapper with fresh herbs and yoghurt, and Steamed green beans (see recipes on pages 197 and 216)

Day 6

Breakfast

1 bowl rolled oats

1 piece wholegrain toast with Omega 3 margarine

Lunch

2 slices smoked salmon with tabouli salad or cottage cheese

Dinner

Pasta with eggplant, and Zucchini stir-fry (see recipes on pages 203 and 226)

Day 7

Breakfast

Dr Walker's super-charged breakfast for G types:

10–15 natural nuts (preferably walnuts, almonds and macadamias)

1–2 dsp LSA (crushed linseeds, sunflower seeds and almonds)
1 heaped dsp unprocessed bran
Combination of blueberries (¼ cup), 2–3 strawberries and ½ banana
150 ml low-fat milk blended with 50–100 g low-fat yoghurt

or

1 fried or boiled egg on 1 piece wholegrain toast
1 glass freshly squeezed juice or 1 cup herbal tea

Lunch

100 g turkey, cranberry sauce, lettuce and 1 slice low-fat cheese on 2 slices wholegrain bread
1 piece fruit

Dinner

Turkey meat loaf, and Baked pumpkin with mushrooms and soy sauce (see recipes on pages 224 and 189)

CHAPTER 14

Recipes

These recipes correspond to the meals suggested in the four body types' seven-day food programs (Chapters 10 to 13). They are listed in alphabetical order.

ASPARAGUS AND POTATO SOUP

A *Recommended for Adrenal body type*

(Serves 4)

2 cups potato, diced
12 asparagus spears
Salt and pepper to season
5 cups vegetable stock

Place ingredients in large saucepan. Bring to the boil and simmer for 30 minutes. Transfer to blender and mix until smooth. Return to saucepan and bring to the boil.

AVOCADO AND CASHEW SALAD

T *Recommended for Thyroid body type*

(Serves 2)

1 avocado, sliced
1 mango, sliced
4 spring onions, sliced
8 cashew nuts
2 tbsp parsley, chopped

Salad dressing

1 clove garlic, crushed
½ cup lemon juice
1 tsp mustard
1 tsp honey

Combine dressing ingredients and drizzle over salad. Serve.

AVOCADO PASTA

G *Recommended for Gonadal body type*

(Serves 4)

1 avocado, halved and stoned
4 shallots, chopped
1 clove garlic, minced
2 tbsp parsley, chopped
Rind and juice of 1 lemon

350 g pasta shells
3 tbsp yoghurt
Black pepper, freshly ground

Cook the pasta and drain. Mash avocado and mix remaining ingredients into it. Combine with pasta and serve.

BAKED PUMPKIN WITH MUSHROOMS AND SOY SAUCE

G *Recommended for Gonadal body type*

(Serves 4)

1 butternut or small pumpkin
1 cup cauliflower, in small pieces
1 cup broccoli, in small pieces
10–12 French beans, cut into 3 cm lengths
3 zucchini, cut into 1 cm thick slices
16–20 snow peas
16–20 button mushrooms, thinly sliced
¾ cup whole blanched almonds, roasted on dry baking tray
½ tsp each turmeric, coriander, ground ginger and cumin
Black pepper
1 tsp soy sauce
2 tsp extra virgin olive oil

Cut pumpkin in half lengthwise and remove seeds. Scoop

out small balls of flesh with spoon, leaving 2 cm of flesh around edge of skin. Place pumpkin skins in ovenproof pan with small quantity of water and bake in moderate oven for 30 minutes, or microwave, until skins are tender. In large saucepan, heat oil and carefully fry spices. Add cauliflower pieces and pumpkin balls together with a little water and cook for 3–4 minutes. Add broccoli, beans and zucchini, stir well and cook for a further 3 minutes. Add snow peas and mushrooms, heat through and stir in soy and pepper. Add roasted almonds, leaving a few aside. Pile vegetables into pumpkin shells, scatter a few almonds over the top, reheat and serve.

BROCCOLI WITH ALMONDS

T *Recommended for Thyroid body type*

(Serves 2)

3 cups broccoli
3 cloves garlic, crushed
3 tbsp flaked almonds
1 tbsp extra virgin olive oil

Heat oil in frying pan and fry garlic. Add broccoli. When cooked, remove from heat, sprinkle with almonds and serve.

CAJUN CHICKEN

C *Recommended for Controller body type*

(Serves 4)

1 kg chicken fillets, thinly sliced
3 egg tomatoes, finely chopped
3 limes
3 shallots, chopped
1 red onion, sliced
1 tin sweet corn kernels
Tomato salsa
¼ cup cajun powder
3 tbsp balsamic vinegar
Extra virgin olive oil

Mix chicken with cajun powder. Add 3 tbsp grated lime rind. Cover and refrigerate for 30 minutes. Cook chicken in frying pan using oil, then add onions and corn kernels. Cook until onion is tender. Mix in tomatoes, shallots, juice from lime, and balsamic vinegar. Serve with salsa as topping.

CAULIFLOWER NEAPOLITAN

C *Recommended for Controller body type*

(Serves 4)

1 large cauliflower head
2 tbsp parsley, chopped

½ cup parmesan cheese, grated
2 cups fresh breadcrumbs
2 tbsp extra virgin olive oil

Cut cauliflower into small pieces. Cook in 2 cups boiling water for about 8 minutes or until tender, then drain in colander. Heat oil in frying pan and fry breadcrumbs. Oil a shallow baking dish, sprinkle it with a little grated parmesan cheese, arrange the cauliflower pieces in the dish and sprinkle with breadcrumbs mixed with remaining parmesan cheese. Put dish in hot oven (230°C/450°F) for 5 minutes or until top is golden. Remove from oven and sprinkle with parsley.

CELERY AND ONION OMELETTE

C *Recommended for Controller body type*

(Serves 1)

½ cup celery, sliced
2 green onions, sliced
2 eggs
2 tsp vegetable oil
1 tsp water

Heat 1 tsp oil in small frying pan. Sauté celery and onions for 4–5 mins until tender, then remove from pan. Beat eggs together with water until mixed. Heat remaining oil in pan and add eggs. Gently stir mixture towards edges of pan until set. Put celery and onion on one half of omelette and fold other half over filling. Slide onto plate.

CHICKEN BURGERS

A *Recommended for Adrenal body type*

(Serves 2)

2 chicken breasts, boned and skinned
½ medium onion, minced
4 large mushrooms
1 egg
2 tbsp dried breadcrumbs
½ tsp salt
1 tsp vegetable oil

Grind chicken in food processor. Add remaining ingredients except mushrooms and oil. Blend and form into four patties. Heat oil in frying pan and cook over medium heat, turning once. Toast mushrooms under grill for 5 minutes. Serve burgers topped with mushrooms.

CORN PANCAKES

C *Recommended for Controller body type*

(Serves 4)

2 cups fresh corn kernels

2 egg yolks
2 egg whites, beaten
2 tbsp plain flour

Combine corn, yolks and flour. Fold in egg whites. Cook together in greased pan.

FRIED WHITE FISH

T *Recommended for Thyroid body type*

(Serves 2)

White fish (1–2 pieces per person)
¼ lemon
Fresh herbs, chopped
Plain flour
Canola or macadamia oil

Dust fish fillets with plain flour. Heat oil in frying pan and add fish. Fry for 2 minutes on each side. Serve with ¼ lemon and boiled new potatoes sprinkled with chopped fresh herbs.

GREEK SALAD WITH RED WINE DRESSING

A *Recommended for all body types*

(Serves 4)

3 cups snow peas, sliced
1 salad onion, sliced
1 cup cherry tomatoes
1 clove garlic, chopped
½ cup black olives, seeded
2 tsp fresh thyme, chopped
1 cup fetta cheese, cubed
1 tbsp red wine dressing (see below)

Combine ingredients, cover and refrigerate.

Red wine dressing

½ tsp garlic, crushed
1 tbsp lime juice
½ cup red wine vinegar
1 tsp Dijon mustard
½ cup macadamia or other oil

Place ingredients in screw-top jar, shake and store in refrigerator.

GRILLED CHICKEN WITH TOMATO SALSA

T *Recommended for Thyroid body type*

(Serves 4)

4 chicken breasts
1 tsp garlic, crushed
2 tsp tumeric
1 cup low-fat natural yoghurt

Salsa

8 tomatoes, diced
1 onion, chopped
1 tbsp parsley, chopped
Juice of 1 lime
2 tsp coriander seeds
Fresh chilli (to flavour)

Mix yoghurt, tumeric and garlic, and brush over chicken. Combine salsa ingredients in serving bowl and refrigerate until needed. Grill chicken on both sides for 7 minutes. Slice and serve with salsa.

GRILLED SNAPPER WITH FRESH HERBS AND YOGHURT

G *Recommended for Gonadal body type*

(Serves 4)

4 fillets snapper or other white fish fillets
2 tbsp each parsley and dill, chopped
Black pepper, freshly ground
8 tbsp natural yoghurt
1 tsp rice flour
4 tbsp tomato paste

Preheat grill. Place fish in oiled ovenproof dish. Mix yoghurt, flour, tomato paste, pepper and half of the herbs. Pour over fish, covering completely. Grill for 4–5 minutes, without turning, until fish is cooked through. Sprinkle with remaining herbs and serve with green salad.

LAMB AND FENNEL KEBABS

T *Recommended for Thyroid body type*

(Serves 4)

400 g lamb fillets, cut into strips
4 long bamboo skewers
1 fennel bulb, diced
1 tbsp fresh dill, chopped
2 tbsp white grape juice
2 tsp extra virgin olive oil

Soak skewers in water to prevent burning. Thread lamb and fennel onto skewers and dip into grape juice. Grill or BBQ, basting with oil, and sprinkle with dill.

LEMON CHICKEN STIR-FRY

C *Recommended for Controller body type*

(Serves 2)

300 g lean, boneless chicken
1 cup each green beans, mushrooms, and carrots, sliced
1 cup broccoli pieces
1 cup fresh bean sprouts
Chopped parsley to garnish
1 tbsp lemon rind, finely grated
3½ tbsp lemon juice
1 tbsp soy sauce
1 tsp honey
1 tbsp cold-pressed canola oil
½ cup water

Cut chicken into pieces then stir-fry in hot oil in large wok for 5 minutes or until cooked through. Remove from wok. Stir-fry carrots and beans until tender but still crunchy. Add bean sprouts, mushrooms and chicken pieces and cook for a few more minutes. Mix lemon rind, lemon juice, soy sauce and water, then add to wok. Heat gently and serve with 1 cup cooked rice or rice noodles. Garnish with parsley and serve.

LEMON SALMON

T *Recommended for Thyroid body type*

(Serves 1)

1 salmon fillet
Handful coriander, chopped
Handful mint, chopped
Juice and zest of 1 lemon
75 g natural yoghurt
1 tbsp apple cider vinegar
Black pepper, freshly ground

Place salmon fillet on ovenproof dish, sprinkle lemon juice and zest over top. Add ground pepper. Grill under medium heat for 10–15 minutes, or until cooked to taste. Make dressing by blending yoghurt, mint and vinegar together. Serve salmon with dressing and garnish with coriander.

LENTIL SOUP

G *Recommended for Gonadal type*

(Serves 4)

4 leeks, chopped
2 carrots, chopped
1 cup lentils
4 cups vegetable stock
Handful mint, chopped, to garnish

Place ingredients in large saucepan, bring to the boil and simmer for 1 hour. Blend vegetables and liquid. Return soup to pan, heat through and serve with garnish.

MAYONNAISE

C *Recommended for Controller body type*

1 large egg
½ tsp salt
1 tsp dry mustard
3 tbsp apple cider vinegar
1¼ cup extra virgin olive oil

Place egg, mustard, vinegar and salt in blender with 2 tbsp oil. Mix for 5–10 seconds and drizzle in remaining oil slowly until mayonnaise consistency is achieved. Store in screw-top jar in fridge until needed.

MEXICAN STUFFED CHICKEN

T *Recommended for Thyroid body type*

(Serves 2)

2 chicken breasts, skinned and boned
2 tbsp mild green chilli, chopped
1 egg, beaten
30 g tasty cheese, cut into 2 slices
1 tbsp parmesan cheese, grated

1 tbsp dried breadcrumbs
½ tsp chilli powder

Preheat oven to 200°C/375°F. Pound chicken breasts until thin. On each breast, place chilli and cheese slice. Roll up and place in baking dish. Brush with egg. Mix together breadcrumbs, parmesan cheese and chilli powder, and sprinkle over chicken, forming a crust. Bake for 20 minutes until crust has browned.

NASI GORENG

A *Recommended for Adrenal body type*

(Serves 2–4)

1 cup prawn pieces
4 spring onions, chopped
1 cup mushrooms, sliced
Cucumber slices and tomato wedges, to garnish
2 tsp ginger, chopped
2 tbsp tomato pasta sauce
4 cups brown Basmati rice, cooked

Combine all ingredients except rice in saucepan, and stir-fry. Add rice and stir. Serve with garnish.

PASTA WITH BROCCOLI, BACON AND CHILLI

A *Recommended for Adrenal body type*

(Serves 4)

100 g bacon, finely chopped
450 g broccoli
½ long red chilli, chopped
Rind of 1 lemon, finely grated
300 g pasta of your choice
Black pepper, freshly ground
1 tbsp extra virgin olive oil
Shaved parmesan cheese to flavour

Boil large saucepan of water, add broccoli and cook for 1 minute. Transfer to bowl of cold water, then chop finely. Reserve 50–100 ml of broccoli stock. Add pasta to fresh boiling water, cook for 12 minutes, then drain. Cook bacon, chilli and garlic in frying pan with extra virgin olive oil until bacon is crisp. Add bacon mixture to pasta with broccoli, lemon, broccoli stock and pepper. Serve with shaved parmesan sprinkled over top.

PASTA WITH EGGPLANT

G *Recommended for Gonadal body type*

(Serves 4)

3 medium eggplants, cut into cubes
1 medium onion, chopped
2 cloves garlic, crushed
440g tin peeled tomatoes (no added salt)
½ tsp oregano
1 tbsp fresh parsley, chopped
Salt and black pepper, freshly ground
250 g penne or shell pasta
1 tbsp tomato puree
1 tsp mustard powder
4 tbsp extra virgin olive oil
Parmesan cheese, grated, to flavour

Place eggplant in colander and sprinkle with salt (to draw out bitter juices). Leave for 30 minutes, rinse thoroughly and pat dry. Cook pasta in boiling water. Rinse in hot water and keep warm. Cook onion and garlic in oil for 5 minutes until onion is tender. Add eggplant, stirring until lightly browned. Add rest of ingredients and simmer gently for 10 minutes until eggplant is cooked through, stirring occasionally. Pour sauce over pasta and serve sprinkled with parmesan cheese.

PEPPERED STEAK

C *Recommended for Controller body type*

(Serves 4)

4 lean fillet steaks (100–125 g each)
Large handful tarragon, chopped
4 tsp black or green peppercorns, crushed
150 ml Greek yoghurt with 1 tsp rice flour added
30 ml brandy
2 tbsp olive oil

Place steaks on crushed peppercorns and press down to encrust the meat on both sides. Heat oil in frying pan and fry steaks for 2 minutes on each side. Reduce heat and cook to taste. Remove steaks from pan. Add brandy to frying pan, remove from heat and set alight. When flame has died down, stir in yoghurt and tarragon, and heat through. Pour sauce over steaks and serve.

PROTEIN BOOST

T *Recommended for Thyroid body type*

(Serves 2)

1 tsp nutmeg or 1 tsp cinnamon
2 eggs
2 cups milk

150 ml low-fat yoghurt
1 tsp vanilla essence
1 tbsp lecithin

Mix all the ingredients in a blender.

PROVENCAL FISH

A *Recommended for Adrenal body type*

(Serves 2–3)

500 g lean fish (sole, flounder or sea bass)
1 clove garlic, crushed
4 fresh tomatoes, peeled and chopped
100 g mushrooms, sliced
1 tsp extra virgin olive oil
pepper, to taste

Preheat oven to 210°C/400°F. Heat oil in frying pan and cook mushrooms for 2–3 minutes. Stir in tomatoes and garlic, then add pepper. Cut fish into 4 pieces and place in shallow baking dish. Cover with tomato mixture. Bake uncovered for 10–15 minutes.

PUMPKIN SOUP

A *Recommended for Adrenal body type*

(Serves 4)

2 cups pumpkin, chopped
1 carrot, chopped
1 leek, chopped
1 tbs extra virgin olive oil
1 tsp caraway seeds
Parsley, chopped, and natural yoghurt, to garnish
5 cups vegetable stock

Stir-fry vegetables in oil for 5–10 minutes in a large pot. Add vegetable stock and caraway seeds. Bring to a slow boil. When vegetables have softened, blend together. Add chopped parsley and natural yoghurt to taste.

QUICK-COOK SALMON OR TUNA

C *Recommended for Controller body type*

(Serves 6)

6 tuna or salmon steaks
1 lemon
Fresh herbs of your choice
¼ cup macadamia or canola oil

Heat frying pan, add oil and lightly fry fish for 3 minutes on each side. Serve with mashed potatoes sprinkled with fresh herbs, and a green salad.

RAW VEGETABLE SALAD

A **G** *Recommended for Adrenal and Gonadal body types*

(Serves 4–6)

Cos lettuce
6 zucchini, finely diced
400 g broccoli, cut into small pieces
3 shallots, finely chopped
400 g stringless green beans, sliced
1 green capsicum, finely sliced
1 red capsicum, finely sliced
4 carrots, sliced
1 ripe avocado, finely sliced
Handful fresh coriander and parsley, finely chopped

SALAD DRESSING

6 cloves garlic, crushed
Juice of 1 lemon
½ cup apple cider vinegar
1 tbsp seed mustard
1 cup extra virgin olive oil

Put salad dressing ingredients into screw-top jar and shake. Tear lettuce leaves into pieces and place in salad bowl. Combine remaining salad ingredients in bowl on top of lettuce. Drizzle dressing over top.

RED KIDNEY BEAN SOUP

T *Recommended for Thyroid body type*

(Serves 4–6)

1 smoked ham hock
1 large carrot
1 stick celery
4 cups red kidney beans
2 x 810 g tin peeled tomatoes (no added salt)
1½ L water

Soak kidney beans overnight. The next day, bring water and ham hock to the boil in large saucepan. Reduce to simmer and cook for 45 minutes, or until flesh is coming off the bone. Remove ham from pan (retain stock), cool and remove skin, bone and fat, keeping pieces of pink meat. Add kidney beans and tomatoes to stock, simmer for 1–2 hours, or until beans are tender, stirring occasionally (add water as necessary). Meanwhile, peel and grate carrot, chop celery (including leaves) and add to soup with meat. Simmer for a further 30 minutes.

SALMON PATTIES

G *Recommended for Gonadal body type*

(Serves 4)

2 cups (210 g) tinned salmon
2 cloves garlic, chopped
2 tbsp parsley, chopped
1 cup rice, cooked
1 egg, beaten
1–2 cups breadcrumbs
extra virgin olive oil

Combine all ingredients except breadcrumbs. Form into patties and coat with breadcrumbs. Fry in extra virgin olive oil for 3–4 minutes each side.

SESAME PRAWNS WITH ASPARAGUS

T *Recommended for Thyroid body type*

(Serves 2)

500 g prawns, peeled and de-veined
1 bunch asparagus, sliced into 1 cm pieces
1 small slice fresh ginger, minced
2 tsp sesame seeds
1 tsp soy sauce
½ tsp cornstarch
1 tsp vegetable oil

Place sesame seeds in wok and toast for 2–3 minutes. Remove from heat. Heat ½ tsp oil in frying pan and fry asparagus for 2 minutes. Remove from pan. Heat remaining oil in frying pan and fry prawns for 3–4 minutes. Add asparagus and cook for further 30 seconds. Stir together soy sauce, ginger and cornstarch and add to frying pan, coat prawns and asparagus. Sprinkle with toasted sesame seeds.

SMOOTHIES

BANANA

C **T** *Recommended for Controller and Thyroid body types*

(Serves 1)

1 banana
1 cup soy milk or n-3 enhanced milk
2 tsp honey

Mix all ingredients in blender.

BERRY

C *Recommended for Controller body type*

(Serves 2)

½ cup blueberries
2 bananas

1 tsp cinnamon
3 scoops frozen yoghurt
1 tsp honey

Mix all ingredients in blender.

SPAGHETTI POMODORI

A *Recommended for Adrenal body type*

(Serves 6–8)

6–8 ripe tomatoes, without skins
2 cloves garlic, finely chopped
1 cup rocket, chopped
Black pepper, freshly ground
1 small tin chickpeas, drained and rinsed
500 g spaghetti
3–4 tbsp extra virgin olive oil

Plunge tomatoes into boiling water for a few minutes and then remove to bowl of cold water. Roughly chop tomatoes and place pieces into serving bowl. Add chickpeas, rocket and garlic, then mix in oil and pepper. Refrigerate for 1 hour, then cook spaghetti. Pour tomato mixture over spaghetti and serve.

SPAGHETTI WITH DICED TOMATOES

G *Recommended for Gonadal body type*

(Serves 4)

10 large garlic cloves, finely sliced
1 kg ripe cherry tomatoes, chopped
20 sun-dried tomatoes
20 black, pitted olives
2 tbsp pine nuts, toasted
100 g rocket
Black pepper, freshly ground
200 g spaghetti
4 tbsp extra virgin olive oil

Cook spaghetti and drain. Return to saucepan. Heat oil in frying pan, add garlic and fry lightly. Remove from heat. Mix warm oil from frying pan, garlic, chopped tomatoes, olives, pepper and then rocket. Gently stir in nuts and serve over spaghetti, with fresh green salad.

SPECIAL BEANS

G *Recommended for Gonadal body type*

(Serves 2–4)

2 tomatoes, cut into wedges
1 cup green peas, cooked
2 tsp fresh ginger, chopped
4 spring onions, sliced

2 cloves garlic, crushed
1 cup bean sprouts
20 pitted black olives
1 zucchini, sliced
2 cups cooked green beans
¼ cup cashew nuts
½ tsp each cumin, coriander and black pepper
1½ tbsp extra virgin olive oil

Heat oil in frying pan and sauté onion, garlic and spices. Add all ingredients and cook until flavours are combined. Serve hot.

SPICY PERCH FILLETS WITH CAPSICUM AND TOMATO SALSA

C *Recommended for Controller body type*

(Serves 4)

4 x 200 g perch fillet
1 small red capsicum, coarsely chopped
1 seeded Lebanese cucumber, coarsely chopped
1 celery stick, trimmed and coarsely chopped
150 g mixed lettuce leaves
2 tbsp lemon juice
¼ cup mild chilli sauce
1 tbsp olive oil

Combine 1 tbsp lemon juice and ¼ cup chilli sauce in

bowl, then rub into skin of each fish fillet. Cook fillets on heated and lightly oiled grill plate (or BBQ) until lightly browned. Cover to keep warm. Make lemon dressing by combining oil, remaining lemon juice and chilli sauce in screw-top jar. Shake well. Place capsicum, cucumber, tomato, celery and half of dressing in bowl. Toss gently to combine. Divide lettuce leaves and fillets between plates. Top fillets with salsa, drizzle lettuce with lemon dressing.

SPICY SALMON STEAK

A *Recommended for Adrenal body type*

(Serves 4)

4 salmon fillets
2 cloves garlic, crushed
Handful coriander, chopped
1 tbsp oregano, chopped
Juice and rind of 1 lemon
½ tbsp paprika
½ tbsp cayenne pepper
½ tbsp cracked pepper
2 tbsp extra virgin olive oil
Natural yoghurt for topping

Mix all marinade ingredients together except for yoghurt. Place salmon in flat dish and pour over marinade. Stand for 30 minutes in fridge. Cook in non-stick pan for 4–5 minutes on each side, or until cooked. Serve with dollop of natural yoghurt.

SPINACH SOUP AND TOFU

C *Recommended for Controller body type*

(Serves 4)

1½ L beef stock
375 g spinach, chopped
1 tbsp root ginger, sliced
1 cake tofu, cubed
1½ tbsp soy sauce

Bring beef stock to the boil. Add all ingredients, simmer for 15 minutes and serve.

SPRING SALAD

T *Recommended for Thyroid body type*

(Serves 4–6)

6 cups mixed lettuce leaves
½ cup green capsicum, diced
½ cup red capsicum, diced
1 avocado, sliced
2 cups fresh mango or papaya, sliced
1 cup pine nuts, browned under grill or in oven
3 tbsp mayonnaise (for home-made mayonnaise, see above)

Combine all ingredients, and sprinkle with pine nuts.

STEAMED GREEN BEANS

G *Recommended for Gonadal body type*

(Serves 4–6)

500 g green beans, ends cut off
2 cloves garlic, finely chopped
1 tbsp parsley, chopped
Salt and black pepper, freshly ground
1 tsp chilli paste
3 tbsp extra virgin olive oil

Steam the beans for 5 minutes. Drain and rinse under cold tap. Place in bowl and add other ingredients. Stand for 30 minutes, then serve.

STEAMED GREENS

T *Recommended for Thyroid body type*

(Serves 4–6)

100 g green beans, sliced
100 g fresh or frozen peas
100 g snow peas
6 asparagus spears
100 g cabbage, shredded, or 2 bunches bok choy, roughly chopped

Dressing

6 cloves garlic, crushed
Juice of 1 lemon
½ cup apple cider vinegar
1 tbsp seed mustard
1 cup extra virgin olive oil

Place dressing ingredients in screw-top jar and shake. Steam vegetables for 10 minutes, tip onto plate and pour ½ cup of dressing over top.

STIR-FRIED CHICKEN

G *Recommended for Gonadal type*

(Serves 2)

1 whole chicken breast, skinned and boned
1 cup asparagus cut into 2 cm lengths
1 tsp extra virgin olive oil

Marinade

2 green onions, sliced
1 slice fresh ginger, minced
2 tsp soy sauce
1 tsp cornstarch

Place marinade ingredients in screw-top jar and shake. Dice chicken breast and place in bowl with marinade.

Heat ½ tsp oil in wok or frying pan. Add vegetables and cook until tender. Remove from pan. Drain marinade from chicken, and keep. Heat remaining oil in pan, add chicken and cook until it turns white. Add vegetables and marinade and toss together until sauce thickens and vegetables are hot.

STIR-FRIED GREEN BEANS

C *Recommended for Controller type*

(Serves 2)

1 cup green beans
pinch salt
1 tsp vegetable oil

Slice beans crosswise into 2 cm lengths. Heat oil in frying pan and add beans. Stir-fry for 3–5 mins, or until beans are just tender. Sprinkle with salt and serve.

STIR-FRIED SPINACH

A *Recommended for Adrenal body type*

(Serves 4)

1 bunch fresh spinach
3 garlic cloves, sliced
2 spring onions, sliced

1 tbsp oyster sauce
1 tbsp extra virgin olive oil
1 tbsp water

Wash spinach well. Heat oil in pan, add garlic, spring onions and spinach. Stir-fry for 1 minute. Mix water with oyster sauce. Pour over vegetables and serve.

STIR-FRIED VEGETABLES

A *Recommended for Adrenal body type*

(Serves 4)

250 g broccoli
250 g green beans
¼ white cabbage or bok choy, finely chopped
6 mushrooms, finely sliced
1 medium zucchini, sliced
250 g cauliflower, in small pieces
1 medium onion, finely chopped
3 cloves garlic, finely chopped
1 piece fresh ginger, grated
1 tbsp peanut oil
1 tbsp light soy sauce
1 tbsp sesame oil

Heat saucepan or wok, add peanut oil, sesame oil, garlic, ginger and onion. Cook over hot flame. Add broccoli, cauliflower, cabbage and beans and stir rapidly for 3–4 minutes. Add zucchini and mushrooms and cook for further 3 minutes. Add soy sauce. Remove from heat and serve.

TABOULI SALAD

G *Recommended for Gonadal body type*

(Serves 2)

2 medium cloves garlic, crushed
4 shallots, finely chopped
2 tomatoes, finely diced
1 small seeded cucumber, finely chopped
1 cup parsley, finely chopped
10–15 mint leaves, finely chopped
¼ cup fresh lemon juice
Black pepper
¼ cup extra virgin olive oil

Combine all ingredients, refrigerate for half an hour and serve.

TASTY FRITTATA

T *Recommended for Thyroid body type*

(Serves 1)

2 eggs
20 ml milk
cracked pepper
½ small leek, chopped

¼ cup chives, chopped
grated cheese

Beat together 2 eggs and combine with small amount of milk in frying pan. Add cracked pepper and stir over heat until scrambled. Add some chopped leek, chopped chives and grated cheese to flavour. Serve on one slice of thick soy and linseed toast.

TERIYAKI LAMB STIR-FRY

C *Recommended for Controller body type*

(Serves 4)

800 g lean lamb strips
2 cloves garlic, crushed
6 green onions, coarsely chopped
1 long, fresh red chilli, seeded, halved and thinly sliced
500 g baby bok choy, quartered
200 g snow peas, trimmed and tailed
⅓ cup teriyaki sauce
¼ cup sweet chilli sauce
2 tsp sesame oil

Heat half the oil in wok or large frying pan. Stir-fry lamb in batches until browned all over. Remove from pan. Heat remaining oil in same wok. Stir-fry onion, garlic and chilli until fragrant. Add bok choy and snow peas. Stir-fry until bok choy just wilts. Return lamb to wok with remaining ingredients and stir-fry until heated through.

THAI BEEF SALAD 1

T *Recommended for Thyroid body type*

(Serves 2)

400 g lean beef fillet steaks, thinly sliced
½ red onion, thinly sliced
1 small cucumber, sliced into strips
150 g cherry tomatoes, halved
100 g rocket
Handful mint, chopped
Handful coriander, chopped
Handful unsalted cashew nuts
1 tbsp extra virgin olive oil

Dressing

1 red chilli, finely chopped
Juice and rind of 1 lime
1 tbsp tomato paste
1 tbsp brown sugar
1 tbsp water

Stir-fry beef in oil until cooked to taste. Place to one side. Mix dressing ingredients together in frying pan and simmer until sugar has dissolved. Remove from heat. Place rocket, onion, cucumber, tomatoes, cashew, mint and coriander in bowl and mix. Top salad with beef slices and drizzle with dressing.

THAI BEEF SALAD 2

A *Recommended for Adrenal body type*

(Serves 4)

800 g lean rump beef steak
3 Lebanese cucumbers, thinly sliced
6 green onions, thinly sliced
150 g bean sprouts
250 g cherry tomatoes, halved
1 cup fresh mint, chopped
1½ cups coriander, chopped
60 ml lime juice
60 ml fish sauce
60 ml sweet chilli sauce
1 tbsp soy sauce

Marinate beef with 2 tbsp fish sauce and 1 tbsp lime juice in bowl, cover and refrigerate for 30 minutes. Drain beef and discard marinade. Cook beef on lightly oiled grill until browned. Slice thinly. Mix cucumber, onion, sprouts, mint, tomatoes and coriander in bowl. Combine remaining fish sauce and lime juice with chilli sauce and soy sauce in screw-top jar and shake well. Add beef and dressing to salad ingredients, toss to combine.

TOFU, LENTIL AND TOMATO SALAD

T **G** *Recommended for Thyroid and Gonadal body types*

(Serves 4)

1 clove garlic, crushed
12 cherry tomatoes
12 sun-dried tomatoes
6 pitted black olives
100 g wild rocket or baby spinach
1 tbsp coriander, chopped
1 tbsp parsely, chopped
11 tbsp lemon juice
Black pepper, freshly ground
75 g green lentils, rinsed, and cooked for 20 minutes
200 g firm tofu, diced into 1 cm cubes
Dash of tabasco sauce
2 tbsp extra virgin olive oil

Preheat grill. Mix lentils, lemon juice, parsley, coriander, olive oil, garlic, tabasco, tomatoes and pepper in bowl. Baste tofu with oil and grill for 1 minute each side.

Place rocket or spinach on plate, divide lentil salad between plates and garnish with olives. Top with tofu and drizzle remaining dressing over top.

TURKEY MEAT LOAF

G *Recommended for Gonadal body type*

(Serves 2–3)

500 g turkey meat, minced
1 onion, diced
6 mushrooms, sliced
½ cup snow peas
1 tbsp tomato paste
¼ cup Basmati rice
1 egg, beaten
3 tbsp low-fat mayonnaise
1 cup hot vegetable or chicken stock

Combine all ingredients except stock. Place mixture in lightly greased loaf tin. Bake at 180°C/350°F for 20 minutes. Cover with hot stock and cook for further 20 minutes, basting frequently.

VEGETARIAN OMELETTE

T *Recommended for Thyroid body type*

(Serves 1)

½ onion, finely sliced
½ tomato
4 mushrooms
2 eggs, beaten

Cracked pepper
Extra virgin olive oil spray

Fry onion in frying pan, in oil. When brown, add tomato and mushrooms. Pour in eggs and add cracked pepper. Let set for 1–2 minutes, then turn.

ZUCCHINI STIR-FRY

G *Recommended for Gonadal body type*

(Serves 2)

2 cloves garlic, crushed
1 cup zucchini, sliced
1 cup tomato, diced
1 cup mushrooms, sliced
2 tsp fresh ginger, grated
½ cup parsley, chopped
2 tsp extra virgin olive oil

Heat oil and lightly fry garlic. Add vegetables and stir-fry, adding water to keep moist. Stir for 2–3 minutes, then serve.

CONCLUSION

Basic principles for all body types

1. Calculate your ideal body weight:
Body Mass Index = weight (kilograms) ÷ height (metres^2)

<20	Underweight
20–26	Normal
26–30	Overweight
>30	Obese
>40	Morbidly obese

If your BMI is 20–26, you are in the ideal range. If your BMI is 26–30, you should aim to lose 5–10 kg. You are considered obese if your BMI is 30–40, and you should make your goal to lose 10–20 kg. If your BMI is greater than 40, you should aim to lose 20 kg.

Please note that these suggested figures for weight loss are purely guidelines and may vary for individuals. In Adrenal types, for example, excess muscle mass will elevate the BMI. (Some high performance athletes have a BMI of 30 with no significant fat load.) The suggested weight loss figures are for a period of 3–6 months.

2. Another useful measurement to take is your waist circumference at the umbilicus. Males should aim for <100cms, and females <89cms.

3. Most diets have a finite time frame. The Dr Walker Lifestyle Program requires lifelong behavioural change and thus it is important to set realistic goals. Simply cutting back on your food intake by around 30 per cent in the initial stages of the program will have a significant impact on your weight and health.

4. Basic hints:

    - use smaller plates
    - eat smaller servings
    - if you have an acute craving, wait 10–15 minutes and if the craving is still there, consume half of what you would normally eat.
    - apples, oranges and mandarins are excellent foods to satisfy cravings and can be eaten at any time.

5. Buy a pedometer and wear it! Aim for at least 10,000 steps daily. See every day and every outing as an opportunity for movement – not an imposition. EVERY STEP COUNTS.

6. All body type groups are encouraged to consume 2–3 pieces of fruit a day, and 3–4 serves of vegetables a day. (The only exception to this is the Thyroid type, who should be consuming only 1 piece of fruit per day and 4–6 serves of vegetables).

7. The Walker 19/21 rule states that for two meals per week you can relax the program. Prohibition never works and is usually a major reason why diets fail.

8. All body types should consume plenty of water throughout the day, in addition to the specific herbal teas suggested for your type.

9. Weigh yourself soon after waking every morning to keep track of your progress.

10. A major life change which will improve the quality and quantity of your life isn't about making one major decision to change. It's about making 30 or 40 small decisions every day – deciding not to eat that cake or that cookie, to have that piece of fruit, to take the stairs rather than the escalator, not to scream at the person who tried to cut in front of you in the traffic. These daily small steps will add up to the success of your program.

Good luck!

Dr Ross Walker

The Cell Factor

Have you noticed that more and more people in our society are constantly tired, gaining weight (despite the health industry's increasingly strident recommendations for low-fat diets), and are stressed beyond belief? Our everyday, modern environment of synthetic and convenience food, technology that reduces physical effort and exercise – from the car you drive to work to the remote control for the television – not to mention the stresses and strains of the corporate and business world are all to blame. But what can we do about it?

Strangely, most people seem to accept this state of affairs, and feel powerless to change their life and health for the better. Yet there is a solution that will ensure a longer, healthier life. The basic unit of function of our bodies are our cells. Once we restore our cells back to good health, our body easily follows suit.

Dr Ross Walker, one of Australia's best-known cardiologists, shows you how to achieve optimum cell health in a book that can literally change your life. *The Cell Factor* demonstrates simple, easy to achieve steps to ensure weight loss, improve energy and, most importantly, improve the quality and quantity of life itself.

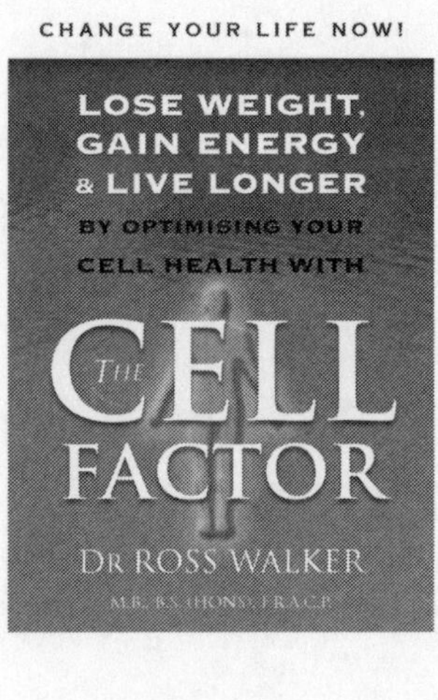

Dr Ross Walker

The Life Factor

Stress, exhaustion, anger and dissatisfaction – these are the banes of modern life. Most of us simply accept them as unavoidable conditions of the world we live in. But we don't have to.

Dr Ross Walker, bestselling author of *The Cell Factor*, has created a series of brilliantly simple, five-step programs that will show you how to become happier, healthier and full of life. From managing stress and becoming more energised, to creating positive patterns of thought and achieving balance in everything you do, *The Life Factor* will help you to establish a more empowering and satisfying style of living.

Using all the experience of twenty years of medical practice and the most up-to-date scientific studies from around the world, as well as his trademark commonsense and humour, Dr Ross Walker has written a book for anyone who has ever suffered from the daily grind of modern living.

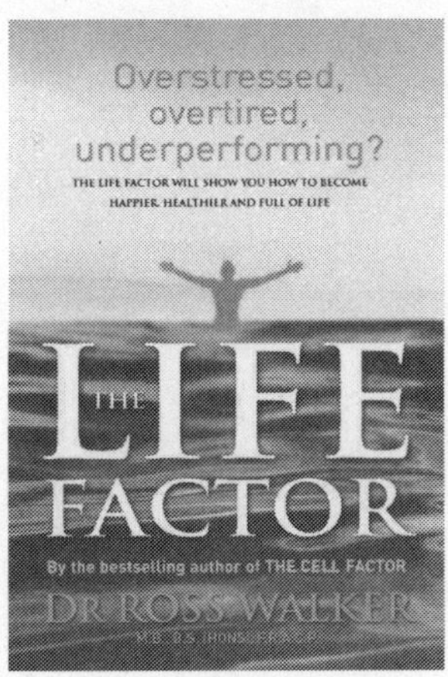